Sexually Transmissible Oral Diseases

Sexually Transmissible Oral Diseases

Editor:

S.R. Prabhu
BDS; MDS (Oral Path); FFDRCSI (Oral Med) FDSRCS(Eng); FDSRCS(Edin);
FDSRCPS (Glas); FFGDPRCS(UK); FICD
Honorary Associate Professor, University of Queensland,
School of Dentistry, Brisbane, Australia

Section Editors:

Nicholas van Wagoner, MD; PhD
Associate Professor of Medicine, Department of Infectious Diseases, UAB
Heersink School of Medicine, Birmingham, Alabama, USA

Jeff Hill, DMD
Professor of Restorative Sciences, UAB School of Dentistry and Director
HIV/AIDS Dental Clinic, Department of Infectious Diseases, UAB
Heersink School of Medicine in Birmingham, Alabama, USA

Shailendra Sawleshwarkar, MD; PhD
Associate Professor, Sexual Health, Sydney Medical School, Faculty of
Medicine and Health, The University of Sydney, Sydney, Australia

WILEY Blackwell

This edition first published 2023
© 2023 by John Wiley & Sons, Ltd.

Registered Office
John Wiley & Sons Ltd, The Atrium, Southern Gate, Chichester, West Sussex, PO19 8SQ, UK

For details of our global editorial offices, customer services, and more information about Wiley products visit us at www.wiley.com.

Wiley also publishes its books in a variety of electronic formats and by print-on-demand. Some content that appears in standard print versions of this book may not be available in other formats.

Library of Congress Cataloging-in-Publication Data

Names: Prabhu, S.R., editor. | van Wagoner, Nicholas, editor. | Hill, Jeff
  DDS, editor. | Sawleshwarkar, Shailendra, editor.
Title: Sexually transmissible oral diseases / editor, S.R. Prabhu ; section
  editors, Nicholas van Wagoner, Jeff Hill, Shailendra Sawleshwarkar.
Description: Chicester, West Sussex, UK ; Hoboken, New Jersey :
  Wiley-Blackwell, 2023. | Includes bibliographical references and index.
Identifiers: LCCN 2022020157 (print) | LCCN 2022020158 (ebook) | ISBN
  9781119826750 (paperback) | ISBN 9781119826767 (adobe pdf) | ISBN
  9781119826774 (epub)
Subjects: MESH: Oral Manifestations | Sexually Transmitted
  Diseases—complications | Dental Care
Classification: LCC RC200.2 (print) | LCC RC200.2 (ebook) | NLM WC 140 |
  DDC 616.95—dc23/eng/20221103
LC record available at https://lccn.loc.gov/2022020157
LC ebook record available at https://lccn.loc.gov/2022020158

Cover image: Courtesy of S.R. Prabhu
Cover design by Wiley

Set in 9.5/12.5pt STIXTwoText by Straive, Chennai, India
Printed and bound by CPI Group (UK) Ltd, Croydon, CR0 4YY

C9781119826750_040123

To Victims of Covid-19 pandemic and all those frontline healthcare workers who are engaged in the fight against the disease with utmost dedication and courage

Contents

Foreword

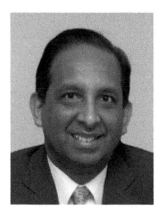

It is a pleasure and a delight for me to pen this message for the inaugural edition of the *'Sexually Transmissible Oral Diseases'* edited by Professor Prabhu.

Even from ancient times it was known that sexually transmitted diseases (STDs) manifested in the mouth. For instance, syphilis and its gummatous manifestations of the oral cavity were known even during Roman times, though the infectivity and presentation of other STDs such as papilloma virus infections leading to oral cancers were a relatively recent finding. These and a plethora of other STDs well described in the book, are now known to manifest intraorally. This comprehensive compendium which brings together the relevant details of all such diseases in a practical, comprehensive and an easily assimilable format, in a single tome is likely to be a wellspring of information for dental practitioners, undergraduate students and postgraduates alike.

The book is timely from three different perspectives. First, due to the sexual promiscuity and the rampant narcotic and drug abuse, there has been an alarming increase in STDs particularly gonorrhoea and syphilis, mainly in the developing world. Second, the gradual realisation that oral health is a key to systemic health, and the importance of the oral-systemic axis by the health professions in general, and finally, the fundamental conceptual realisation that dentists are not only oral surgeons but also oral physicians who are able to advice, diagnose, care and prevent systemic diseases through a number of avenues available to them including the rapidly developing field of salivomics. Such expanded repertoire of dentistry means a deeper understanding of aetiopathogenesis of common STDs, and hence, this book will be a welcome addition to the libraries of all dental practitioners and dental schools.

In closing, I wish to congratulate the team led by Professor Prabhu, for this excellent initiative that fills a relatively big void in the oral medicine and pathology literature and wish the book the success it so well deserves. It will be essential reading for all young practitioners, in particular, who will step into a transformative world where dentists play a key role in delivering general as well as oral healthcare.

Lakshman Samaranayake
DSc (hc), FRCPath, DDS (Glas), FDSRCS (Edin), FRACDS,
FDS RCPS, FHKCPath, FCDSHK
**Professor Emeritus (Microbiomics),
and Immediate-past Dean**
Faculty of Dentistry, The University of
Hong Kong, Hong Kong
Editor-in-Chief, International *Dental Journal of*
the FDI World Dental Federation

May 2022

Preface

Oral manifestations are a common feature of some sexually transmitted diseases (STDs). In such situations, the majority of patients have no knowledge of the possible link between underlying sexually acquired diseases and their presenting oral signs or symptoms. It is also likely that dental practitioners who treat these patients lack adequate knowledge of links between the underlying diseases and their oral presentation. It is important, therefore, that dental practitioners have adequate knowledge of the nature of STDs, their clinical presentations, progression, and impact upon oral and systemic health. They will need, in consultation with the patient's physician, to provide appropriate management of the oral condition.

The extant literature contains a number of case reports and review articles dealing with oral manifestations of some STDs but a single source that provides a comprehensive account of oral manifestations of a wide range of these diseases is not available. Textbooks on oral diseases and on oral medicine do not always deal with STDs in detail. *Sexually Transmissible Oral Diseases* aims to fill this gap by providing oral healthcare providers with a single source designed to be useful in everyday practice. The main purpose of this book is to improve competence of dental practitioners in the recognition and management of oral manifestations of STDs. The book is structured to help dental and medical practitioners work closely, with a holistic approach, in caring for their patients.

This book has 18 chapters grouped in three sections. The first provides an overview including the global STD burden, its impact of on public health and the role of healthcare professionals in the prevention of STDs. Section 2 deals with oral and genital mucosa with respect to their structure and associated microbiota, and highlights the impact of risky sexual behaviours such as oral sex on oral and general health. Section 3 provides detailed information on the oral manifestations of sexually transmissible diseases and those opportunistic infections and neoplasms commonly encountered in human immunodeficiency virus (HIV) disease. Though oropharyngeal infectious mononucleosis and oral candidosis are not primarily sexually transmitted, they are included in Section 3 because of their frequent co-presentation.

We believe this book is the first of its kind targeted at oral healthcare professionals worldwide. This multi-author work has contributors drawn from many parts of the world with expertise in infectious diseases, community medicine, sexual health, dermatology, oral pathology, microbiology and clinical oral medicine. Editor, section editors and chapter contributors hope that this publication will contribute to the missions of global organisations such as the FDI World Dental Federation, the World Health Organisation, Centres for Disease Control and Prevention, and the International Association of Dental Research in promoting health through oral health.

We believe that this publication is a timely addition to the world's dental and medical literature and will be of value to dentists, oral health therapists, dental hygienists, undergraduate and postgraduate dental students, medical practitioners, dermatologists and other healthcare providers.

May 2022

Editor:
S.R. Prabhu, Brisbane
Section Editors:
Nicholas van Wagoner, Alabama
Jeff Hill, Alabama
Shailendra Sawleshwarkar
Sydney

Acknowledgements

I wish to thank Professor Emeritus Lakshman Samaranayake for recognising the potential contribution of this book to general health through oral health and writing a foreword. I am greatly indebted to Associate Professor Nicholas van Wagoner, Professor Jeff Hill and Associate Professor Shailendra Sawleshwarkar for their valuable advice and editorial assistance. I wish to thank distinguished contributors from different parts of the world for their chapter contributions during the challenging times of the Covid-19 pandemic. My sincere thanks are also to those who have shared their clinical and photomicrographic images and enhanced the quality of chapters. We have made every effort to acknowledge the copyrighted material for the pictures used. If copyright infringement has occurred unintentionally, I wish to tender my apologies. Guidance and editorial assistance from the staff of John Wiley & Sons (UK) are gratefully acknowledged.

I wish to acknowledge the unconditional support offered by my wife, Uma Prabhu, during the Covid-19 work from home period during which a significant part of this book was carried out.

May 2022

S.R. Prabhu
Editor

List of Contributors

Amanda Oakley
Dermatologist
Waikato District
Health Board and Adjunct
Associate Professor
Department of Medicine
University of Auckland
New Zealand

Ana L.O.C. Roza
Department of Oral Diagnosis
Piracicaba Dental School
Universidade Estadual de Campinas
Piracicaba
Brazil

Andrea B. Moleri
Department of Oral Medicine
School of Dentistry
Universidade Federal Fluminense
Niterói
Brazil

Anura Ariyawardana
Associate Professor
School of Medicine and Dentistry
Griffith University, Gold Coast
College of Medicine and Dentistry
James Cook University, Cairns
Clinical Principal
Metro South Oral Health
Queensland Health, Brisbane
Australia

Chythra R. Rao
Associate Professor
Department of Community Medicine
Kasturba Medical College
Manipal
India

David H. Felix
Postgraduate Dental Dean and
Director of Dentistry
NHS Education for Scotland
Edinburgh and Honorary Professor
School of Medicine Dentistry and Nursing
University of Glasgow
UK

Henry Fan
Menzies Health Institute Queensland &
School of Medicine and Dentistry
Griffith University
Gold Coast
Australia

Jeff Hill
Professor of Restorative Sciences
UAB School of Dentistry and Director
HIV/AIDS Dental Clinic
Department of Infectious Diseases
UAB Heersink School of Medicine in
Birmingham, Alabama
USA

Jeremy Lau
Registrar Oral Medicine
University of Western Australia
Dental School
Perth
Australia

Mário J. Romañach
Department of Oral Diagnosis and
Pathology
School of Dentistry
Universidade Federal do Rio de Janeiro
Rio de Janeiro
Brazil

Newell W. Johnson
Professor Emeritus
Menzies Health Institute Queensland &
School of Medicine and Dentistry
Griffith University
Gold Coast
Australia

Nicholas van Wagoner
Associate Professor of Medicine
Department of Infectious Diseases
UAB, Heersink School of Medicine
Birmingham
Alabama
USA

Norman Firth
Adjunct Associate Professor
University of Queensland School of
Dentistry
Brisbane, Australia
and
Oral Medicine Specialist Capital and Coast
District Health Board
Wellington
New Zealand

Pallavi Hegde
Senior Resident
Department of Dermatology
Kasturba Medical College
Manipal
India

Raghavendra Rao
Professor and Head
Department of Dermatology
Kasturba Medical College
Manipal
India

Ramesh Balasubramaniam
Associate Professor
University of Western Australia
Dental School
Perth
Australia

S.R. Prabhu
Honorary Associate Professor
University of Queensland
School of Dentistry
Brisbane
Australia

Samuel Sprague
Menzies Health Institute Queensland &
School of Medicine and Dentistry
Griffith University
Gold Coast
Australia

Shailendra Sawleshwarkar
Associate Professor
Sexual Health, Sydney Medical School
Faculty of Medicine and Health
The University of Sydney
Sydney, Australia

Sue-Ching Yeoh
Oral Medicine Specialist
The Chris O'Brien Life house
Camperdown NSW
Australia

Sujitha Reddy
Junior Resident
Department of Dermatology
Kasturba Medical College
Manipal
India

Vidya Pai
Professor
Department of Microbiology
Yenepoya Medical College
Mangaluru
India

Vijayasarathi Ramanathan
Lecturer in Sexual Health
Faculty of Medicine and Health
The University of Sydney
Sydney
Australia

Yasmin Hughes
Registrar, Western Sydney Sexual
Health Centre
Western Sydney Local Health District
Parramatta
New South Wales
Australia

Glossary

Ab	antibody
Ag	antigen
AIDS	Acquired immune deficiency syndrome
ALT	alanine aminotransferase or alanine transaminase
ANA	antinuclear antibody
Anilingus	oro-anal sex
Anti-HAV IgM	antibody to HAV IgM – signifies recent exposure to HAV
Anti-HAV IgG	antibody to HAV IgG – signifies past exposure to HAV or successful vaccination
Anti-HBIgM	antibody to hepatitis B core antigen – signifies recent exposure to HBV
Anti-HBc IgG	antibody to hepatitis B core antigen – signifies past exposure to HBV
Anti-HBe	antibody to hepatitis Be antigen
Anti-HBs	antibody to hepatitis B surface antigen - associated with non-replicative phase or successful vaccination
Anti-HCV	antibody for HCV – indicates infection with HCV has occurred
Anti-HDV	IgG and IgM antibody to the hepatitis D virus
APTT	activated partial thromboplastin time
ART	antiretroviral therapy
ASMA	anti-smooth muscle antibody
AST	aspartate aminotransferase
AZT	azidothymidine, also called zidovudine
B-cell	a type of immune cell
Balanitis	inflammation of the glans penis
Balanoposthitis	vinflammation of the glans penis and the prepuce (foreskin)
BBV	blood-borne virus
BCG	Bacille Calmette-Guerin (tuberculosis vaccine)
Bd	bid twice daily

BV	bacterial vaginosis, a common complex syndrome resulting in a change in the vaginal ecosystem with raised vaginal pH; often asymptomatic but sometimes associated with an abnormal vaginal discharge
CAH	chronic active hepatitis
cART	combination antiretroviral therapy
C & S	culture and sensitivity
CCR5	chemokine co-receptor on the surface of cells which may be used in HIV-cell fusion CD4 cell a helper T-cell which carries the CD4 surface antigen. CD4 cells are the primary target of HIV and CD4 cell numbers decline during HIV disease
CD8	cell a killer or cytotoxic T-cell which carries the CD8 surface antigen
Chancre	the painless ulcer of primary syphilis
Chancroid	a tropical STI caused by *Haemophilus ducreyi*
CIN	cervical intraepithelial neoplasia
Circumcision	removal of the prepuce (foreskin)
CMV	cytomegalovirus
Condylomata acuminata	genital warts
Condylomata lata	moist warty growths occurring in perineum in secondary syphilis
Contact tracing	the following-up, diagnosis and (where possible) treatment of all sexual partners of a patient infected with an STI. Also called 'partner notification'
CRP	C-reactive protein
CT	computed tomography
Cunnilingus	oral sex – mouth to vulva
DGI	disseminated gonococcal infection
DILI	drug-induced liver injury
Dipping	vaginal or anal sex without a condom for varying periods of time prior to ejaculation, i.e. the condom is only applied when the insertive partner is getting near ejaculation
DNA cccDNA	deoxyribonucleic acid covalently closed circular DNA
Donovanosis	a rare STI of great chronicity causing considerable destruction of genital structures if untreated.
DRE	digital rectal examination
EBV	Epstein–Barr virus
EIA	enzyme immunoassay: an immunoassay in which an enzyme, such as a peroxidase is used as a marker to indicate the presence of specific antigens or antibodies (as in treponemal EIA, a specific serological test for syphilis)
ELISA	enzyme linked immunosorbent assay
Epididymo-orchitis	inflammation of epididymis primarily, spreading secondarily to testis

FBC	full blood count
FDA	US Food and Drug Administration
Fellatio	oral sex – mouth to penis
Fisting sexual act	where fist and forearm are inserted into vagina or ano-rectum
Fomites materials	(e.g. towels, sheets etc) which, once contaminated with a microbiological or virological agent, allow transmission of that infection to another individual
FTA-ABS	fluorescent treponemal antibody absorbed serology test, a specific serological test for syphilis
Genital herpes	infection of ano-genital region with sexually transmitted HSV-1 or HSV-2
Genital warts	exophytic clinical manifestation of sexually transmitted ano-genital HPV infection
GGT	gamma glutamyl transferase
GI	gastrointestinal
GIT	gastrointestinal tract
GP	general practitioner
gp120	glycoprotein on the surface of HIV which binds to the CD4 receptor
gp41	glycoprotein on the surface of HIV involved in fusion between HIV and the CD4 cell
GUD	(ano)-genital ulcerative disease
HAART	highly active antiretroviral therapy
HAV	hepatitis A virus
HAVAb	hepatitis A antibody test (IgM or IgG)
HBcAb	see anti-HBc
HBcAg	hepatitis B core antigen
HBeAb	see anti-HBe
HBeAg	HBV 'e' antigen – a marker of viral replication and infectivity
HBIG	hepatitis B immunoglobulin
HBsAg	hepatitis B surface antigen – a marker of current infection which persists in individuals who become carriers
HBsAb	see anti-HBs
HBV	hepatitis B virus
HCC	hepatocellular carcinoma
hCG	human chorionic gonadotropin
HCV	hepatitis C virus
HDV	hepatitis D virus
HHV-8	human herpesvirus-8 – associated with Kaposi's sarcoma
HIV	human immunodeficiency virus
HPV	human papillomavirus
HSIL	high grade squamous intraepithelial lesion
HSV	herpes simplex virus

HVS	high vaginal swab
IDU	injecting drug user
IFN	interferon
Ig	immunoglobulin
INR	international normalised ratio – a test of blood clotting
IRIS	immune reconstitution inflammatory syndrome
IV	intravenous
IVD	*in vitro* diagnostic medical devices
IU	international unit(measurement)
KS	Kaposi's sarcoma
Latency	the situation where an infection enters a quiescent asymptomatic phase and is only detectable by appropriate testing
LFT	liver function test
LGV	lymphogranuloma venereum - a tropical STI caused by *C. trachomatis* serovars L1–L3, now becoming endemic among highly sexually active men who have sex with men
LSIL	low grade squamous intraepithelial lesion
μl	microlitre
ml	millilitre
mmol	millimole
MRI	magnetic resonance imaging
MSM	men who have sex with men
NAAT	nucleic acid amplification test
NNRTI	non-nucleoside reverse transcriptase inhibitor
NPEP	non-occupational post-exposure prophylaxis
NRTI	nucleoside / nucleotide reverse transcriptase inhibitor
NSU	nonspecific urethritis - urethritis where exhaustive laboratory testing fails to find a specific cause (a non-gonococcal, non-chlamydial, non-herpetic, non-trichomonal urethritis)
OCP	ova, cysts, and parasites - looked for on microscopy of faecal specimens
OI	opportunistic infection
Oral sex	use of the mouth in sexual activity (i.e. anilingus, cunnilingus or fellatio)
p24	a core HIV protein
Pathogenicity	the ability of a micro-organism to cause disease in its host
PCP	Pneumocystis pneumonia, also known as Pneumocystis jiroveci pneumonia
PCR	polymerase chain reaction
PEP	post-exposure prophylaxis
pg/ml	picogram per millilitre
PH	primary HIV infection
PI	protease inhibitor

PID	pelvic inflammatory disease
Pili	hair like appendages found on the surface of some bacteria (especially *N. gonorrhoeae*)
PMTCT	preventing mother-to-child transmission of HIV
POCT	point of care testing
PrEP	pre-exposure prophylaxis
Prepuce	foreskin
Proctitis	inflammation of rectal mucosa
Pubic lice	an infestation of body and pubic hair caused by *Pthirus pubis*, usually sexually transmitted in adults
PWID	people who inject drugs
Qd	once daily
Qds, qid	four times daily
RF	rheumatoid factor
Rimming	anilingus, oro-anal sex
RNA	ribonucleic acid
RPR	rapid plasma reagin test – a non-specific quantitated serological test for syphilis
RT	reverse transcriptase
Scabies	skin infestation caused by Sarcoptes scabiei, often sexually transmitted in adults
Screening	testing for the presence of an asymptomatic condition in an apparently healthy individual
Seroconversion	process whereby a serological test for a given microbiological or virological agent changes from non-reactive to reactive, coinciding with recent infection
Serology	diagnostic identification of antibodies (usually), sometimes antigens, in serum
Serovar	group of closely related microorganisms distinguished by a characteristic set of antigen
STI	any infection which is mainly transmitted from one individual to another by sexual activity

Section 1

Sexually Transmitted Diseases: A Global Issue

1

Sexually Transmitted Diseases: An Overview

Yasmin Hughes[1] and Shailendra Sawleshwarkar[2]

[1]Western Sydney Sexual Health Centre, Western Sydney Local Health District, Parramatta, New South Wales, Australia
[2]Sexual Health, Sydney Medical School, Faculty of Medicine and Health, University of Sydney, Sydney Australia

Introduction

Sexually transmitted infections (STIs) spread predominantly by sexual contact, including vaginal, anal and oral sex. Some STIs can also be transmitted from mother to child during pregnancy, childbirth and breastfeeding. The World Health Organisation (WHO) report reveals that more than 30 different bacteria, viruses and parasites are known to be transmitted through sexual contact. Eight of these pathogens are linked to the greatest burden of sexually transmitted disease (STD). Of these STIs, bacterial infections such as syphilis, gonorrhoea, chlamydia and trichomoniasis, a protozoal infection, are currently curable, whereas viral infections such as herpes simplex virus (HSV), human immunodeficiency virus (HIV), human papilloma virus (HPV) and hepatitis B virus infections are incurable [1].

Diagnosis of STIs requires a detailed history, thorough clinical examination, and appropriate investigations. Since many STIs are asymptomatic, screening for common STIs in at-risk populations, regardless of symptoms, is important for STI control and to prevent onward transmission.

Bacterial STIs

Syphilis

Syphilis is an STI caused by the spirochete bacterium, *Treponema pallidum*. The spirochete is transmitted by direct contact with an infectious lesion, gaining access through microabrasions in the skin during vaginal, anal and oral sex. Syphilis earned the name of 'the great imitator' due to its vast array of clinical presentations, including many oral manifestations, which may mimic other conditions. The infection progresses through clinical stages,

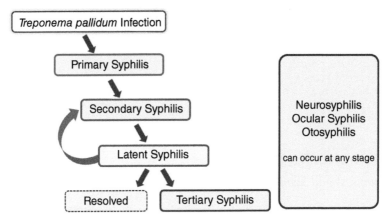

Figure 1.1 Natural history and clinical staging of syphilis. Source: Reproduced with permission from Spach and Mirchandani [2].

known as primary, secondary, latent and tertiary syphilis (Figure 1.1) [2]. The primary, secondary and tertiary phases have all been associated with oral lesions. It is therefore prudent for oral health practitioners to be familiar with the natural history of this infection and its associated oral manifestations.

Epidemiology
Syphilis continues to cause morbidity and mortality worldwide. WHO estimates that 7.1 million new cases of syphilis occurred among adolescents and adults aged 15–49 years worldwide in 2020 [1, 3].

Bacteriology, Risk Factors and Transmission
The etiologic agent in syphilis is *T. pallidum*. *Treponema* belongs to the spirochete class and is a corkscrew-shaped, motile microaerophilic bacterium that requires a live rabbit-model system for culture and cannot be viewed by normal light microscopy. This spirochete bacterium is thin (0.1–0.18 μm in diameter) and 6–20 μm in length with typical corkscrew motion on dark-field microscopy (Figure 1.2) [2, 4].

The major routes of transmission for *T. pallidum* are sexual (during the primary and secondary stages of syphilis) and haematogenous (in utero via transplacental spread to a foetus) [2, 5]. During sexual transmission, *T. pallidum* enters the body via breaches in skin and mucous membranes. Although sexual transmission of *T. pallidum* usually results from contact at genital mucous membranes, it can also occur at other body areas, including the mouth, anorectal areas and cutaneous lesions. Maternal transmission predominantly occurs via transplacental passage of *T. pallidum* during maternal spirochetemia; less often, transmission can occur if the newborn has contact with maternal genital lesions at the time of delivery [2, 5].

Clinical Features
Primary Syphilis
Primary syphilis occurs around the time of initial infection with *T. pallidum* when it penetrates the mucosa, forming an infectious lesion, the chancre, at the site of inoculation within 9–90 days. The lesion is typically a painless, but may be painful, firm, round

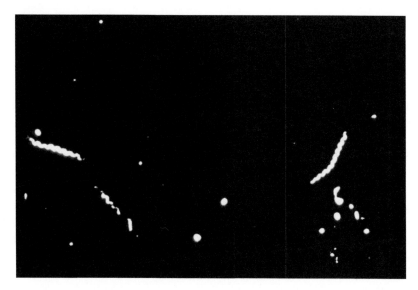

Figure 1.2 *Treponema pallidum*: dark-field microscopy. This photomicrograph shows the typical spiralled 'corkscrew' appearance of several *T. pallidum* spirochetes with the dark-field microscopy technique. Source: Renelle Woodall, 1969, Center for Disease Control (CDC) – PHIL/Public domain.

indurated ulcer lasting from approximately three to seven weeks, which heals without scarring. They may be single or multiple ulcers and occur on the genitalia or other sites of contact such as extra genital sites including the lips, tongue and oral mucosa (see Chapter 12). These lesions are highly infectious and may go unnoticed by the patient before they heal. Left untreated, the infection enters the second stage.

Secondary Syphilis
Within 10 weeks of inoculation, haematogenous and lymphatic spread of the spirochetes may result in clinical features of secondary syphilis, which can affect every system including the central nervous system. Patients with secondary syphilis may present with an array of non-specific features including fever, generalised lymphadenopathy and non-pruritic rash, typically affecting the palms of the hands and soles of the feet. Oral lesions occur in a third of cases of secondary syphilis and can be diverse and non-specific. These include pharyngitis, glistening plaques and oral ulcers [6] (see Chapter 12). The classical lesion, known as the mucous patch, is a shallow, irregular grey-white plaque with an erythematous base. They are usually bilateral, often involving the tongue and may extend to 1 cm in diameter. Snail track ulcers describe multiple mucous patches becoming confluent [6].

Latent Syphilis
Latent syphilis is a stage of syphilis characterised by the persistence of *T. pallidum* organisms in the body without causing signs or symptoms [2]. Clinical signs and symptoms of secondary syphilis may resolve spontaneously, and, if left untreated, the infection enters a latent phase. Patients with latent syphilis typically remain infectious for the first two years of infection, termed early latent, followed by late latent syphilis of variable duration which

is usually non-infectious. While some patients will remain in the latent phase, a third of patients undiagnosed and untreated will enter the tertiary phase, which may occur decades after the initial infection [7].

Tertiary Syphilis

Without treatment, approximately 30% of patients will progress to the tertiary stage at 2–50 years after the original infection [2, 7, 8]. Lesions of tertiary syphilis manifest as locally destructive granulomatous lesions with a necrotic central core affecting the skin, mucous membranes, neural tissue, bone and/or any visceral organ. Oral gummata are rare but may affect the tongue or palate and may range in size to more than 1 cm (see Chapter 12). Perforations of the nasal cavity or the maxillary sinus may complicate palatal gummata [9]. Tertiary syphilis can present as an interstitial glossitis where the tongue appears erythematous with a loss of surface papillae and can become fissured and lobulated [9]. If there is any suspicion of syphilis in a patient presenting for dental care, referral to a medical healthcare provider is necessary. Dental treatment should be deferred, and reasonable infectious disease precautions taken as syphilitic lesions in the first and second stages of disease are highly infectious.

Congenital Syphilis

T. pallidum can be transferred via the placenta from an infected mother to the developing foetus in utero. Untreated syphilis in pregnancy is associated with poor obstetric outcomes including foetal and neonatal death, and congenital syphilis [10, 11]. Clinical manifestations of congenital syphilis include perforation of the hard palate and Hutchinson's triad consisting of interstitial keratitis, vestibulocochlear nerve deafness and Hutchinson teeth. Developmental processes of enamel-forming cells are hindered by *T. pallidum* [12]. Later, formation of the crowns is disrupted, with characteristic semilunar notches on the incisal edges (Hutchinson teeth) [13] (see Chapter 12). Malformation of the enamel of permanent molars results in mulberry molars and doming of the first permanent molars causes Moon's molars. Congenital syphilis may also lead to premature loss of deciduous teeth with resultant delay in speech development and problems with eating [9]. If a child is suspected of having congenital syphilis, referral to a paediatrician with an interest in infectious disease is urgently required.

Diagnosis

Diagnosis of syphilis relies on detailed history, including a sexual history, clinical examination and laboratory investigations. As *T. pallidum* is too fragile for an organism to be cultured, diagnosis is made by direct visualisation of the organism or indirect evidence of infection. For primary chancres, dark ground or dark-field microscopy may be performed, in specialised centres, on exudate obtained from the lesion for direct visualisation of the spirochete. When this is not available, and for cases of secondary syphilis, where lesions are often dry, laboratory diagnosis relies on nucleic acid amplification testing (NAAT) of DNA extracted from infectious lesions and on serological testing of syphilis antibodies. Direct methods have the advantage, in some cases, of detecting infection before a patient has mounted a measurable antibody response that results in a reactive serology result. Serological tests are of two types: treponemal tests and non-treponemal tests. Treponemal tests include syphilis enzyme immunoassay (EIA), *T. pallidum* haemagglutination (TPHA) or fluorescent treponema antibody (FTA) tests, which are specific for *T. pallidum*. FTA is the most sensitive test for detecting early disease. Treponemal serology remains reactive for life and cannot, therefore, be used to distinguish between new and past infections. Non-treponemal tests include Venereal Diseases Research Laboratory (VDRL) or rapid plasma reagin (RPR) which are non-specific cardiolipin antibody tests. Non-treponemal tests are used to identify reinfection or/and to monitor response to treatment. RPR and VDRL are reported as a 'titre'; a high titre is a marker of disease activity with titres reducing with successful treatment. False-positive test results can occur with non-treponemal tests due to other conditions such as hepatitis, infectious mononucleosis, collagen diseases (e.g. systemic lupus erythematosus), pregnancy or ageing. Gummata of tertiary syphilis are diagnosed by clinical evaluation including biopsy and demonstration of *T. pallidum* using silver staining. Patients with confirmed gumma should be screened for other complications of tertiary syphilis including neurosyphilis, ocular syphilis and cardiovascular complications.

Treatment
Penicillin G, administered parenterally, is the preferred drug for treating all stages of syphilis. The preparation(s) of penicillin used (e.g. benzathine, aqueous procaine or aqueous crystalline), the dosage and the length of treatment depend on the stage and clinical manifestations of the disease [2]. A single intramuscular injection of long-acting benzathine penicillin G (2.4 million units administered intramuscularly) will cure a person who has primary, secondary or early latent syphilis. Three doses of long-acting benzathine penicillin G (2.4 million units administered intramuscularly) at weekly intervals are recommended for individuals with late latent syphilis or latent syphilis of unknown duration [14]. Neurosyphilis as well as ocular and otosyphilis is treated with aqueous crystalline penicillin G 18–24 million units per day for 10–14 days (administered intravenously) [14].

Chlamydia

Chlamydia is an STI caused by the bacterium *Chlamydia trachomatis,* an obligate intracellular pathogen which depends entirely on the host cell's adenosine triphosphate for its energy [15]. The bacterium infects columnar epithelium at mucosal sites. Transmission of *C. trachomatis* occurs during ano-rectal sexual intercourse; however, transmission during oral sex and autoinoculation to cause conjunctivitis can occur.

Epidemiology
Chlamydia is the most prevalent bacterial STI in the world. Based on the STI surveillance from WHO, global estimation of new chlamydia cases in 2020 was 129 million [1, 3].

Aetiology/Risk Factors/Transmission
C. trachomatis is an obligate intracellular bacterium with a cell wall and ribosomes similar to those of Gram-negative organisms [16]. Sexually acquired *C. trachomatis* is highly transmissible with adolescents and young adults at increased risk for infection. Risk factors associated with acquisition of chlamydial infection include recent partner change,

multiple sexual partners, past history of STI and unprotected sexual intercourse. Transmission of *C. trachomatis* can also occur from mother to infant via the genital tract during birth [17].

Clinical Features

C. trachomatis causes a wide range of clinical manifestations and complications, including cervicitis, urethritis, pelvic inflammatory disease (PID), tubal infertility, pelvic pain and perihepatitis in women, and urethritis and epididymo-orchitis in men. Other manifestations in men and women may include conjunctivitis, oropharyngeal infection, proctitis/proctocolitis and reactive arthritis. Infants born to mothers with untreated *C. trachomatis* infection may develop conjunctivitis, pneumonia and urogenital infection [17]. Complications of such as epididymitis and epididymo-orchitis may result in men and PID from untreated ascending infection from the cervix in women. A different serovar of *C. trachomatis* can cause lymphogranuloma venereum, which presents as genital ulceration, lymphadenopathy and/or proctitis.

There are no specific oral manifestations of chlamydial infection, but asymptomatic infection of the throat occurs in those performing oral sex [18]. Oropharyngeal infection with *C. trachomatis* is most frequently asymptomatic in both men and women. It can also present as acute tonsillitis, acute pharyngitis or abnormal pharyngeal sensation syndrome (see Chapter 16). When clinical signs and symptoms are described, the presentation can range from minimally symptomatic disease (i.e. dry or pruritic throat) to exudative tonsillopharyngitis. Chlamydial tonsillopharyngitis is marked by generalised pharyngeal and tonsillar hyperaemia with possible addition of swollen anterior pillars and uvula, as well as diffuse purulent exudate on the tonsils [17].

Diagnosis

The *C. trachomatis* cell wall is unique in that it contains an outer lipopolysaccharide membrane but lacks peptidoglycan, meaning that conventional Gram staining is not useful in its detection. Diagnosis of *C. trachomatis* relies on nucleic acid amplification of DNA detected from anogenital or oropharyngeal specimens using NAAT. In most circumstances, the preferred diagnostic method for chlamydial infection is with a *C. trachomatis* NAAT, on urine samples, rectal and throat samples, clinician-collected endocervical and urethral samples, and self-collected vaginal swabs. Pharyngeal sampling is used to screen those who are at risk of asymptomatic throat infection [17]. The clinical significance of oropharyngeal *C. trachomatis* infection is unclear, and prevalence is low, even among populations at high risk. However, when gonorrhoea testing is performed at the oropharyngeal site, chlamydia test results might be reported because certain NAATs detect both bacteria from a single specimen.

Treatment

The recommended first-line treatment of chlamydial infections in non-pregnant women and all men is with a *doxycycline*, 100 mg twice daily, for seven days, with an alternative treatment option of single-dose *azithromycin* [14].

Gonorrhoea

Gonorrhoea is an STI caused by *Neisseria gonorrhoeae,* a Gram-negative bacterium that infects the columnar epithelium of the lower genital tract, rectum, pharynx and conjunctiva [15].

Epidemiology

In 2020, the WHO estimated the pooled global prevalence of urogenital gonorrhoea to be 0.8% in women and 0.7% in men, and in 2020, there were an estimated 82 million gonorrhoea cases worldwide [3].

Bacteriology, Pathogenesis and Transmission

N. gonorrhoeae is a Gram-negative kidney-bean-shaped coccus bacterium that is divided by binary fission and thus usually appears as pairs (diplococci) (Figure 1.3) [19]. The organism is able to attach itself to epithelial cells via several structures located on its surface, allowing it to infect mucosal surfaces, such as the urogenital epithelium, oropharyngeal tract and conjunctival tissue [20, 21]. It also has several virulence factors that facilitate immune evasion [20, 21]. Infection with *N. gonorrhoeae* generates limited immunity allowing repeated infections in an individual [22]

Transmission of *N. gonorrhoeae* can occur from the urethra in a person with gonorrhoea to the vagina or rectum, the vagina or rectum in a person with gonorrhoea to the urethra in a person without gonorrhoea, anogenital tract of a person with gonorrhoea to the pharynx of a person without gonorrhoea or via oral–genital or oral–anal contact; and from the pharynx of a person with gonorrhoea to the urethra of a person without gonorrhoea during fellatio [19]. Perinatal transmission (from mother to infant) can occur during vaginal delivery when a mother with gonorrhoea has not been treated during the perinatal period.

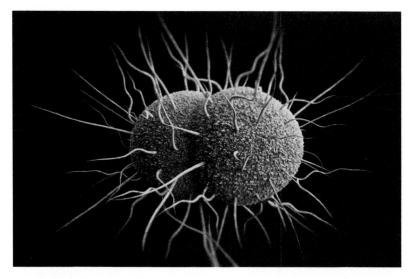

Figure 1.3 *Neisseria gonorrhoeae* [19]. Source: James Archer, 2013, Center for Disease Control (CDC) – PHIL/Public domain.

Clinical Features

N. gonorrhoeae infection may result in diverse clinical syndromes, including urethritis, cervicitis, pharyngitis, proctitis and conjunctivitis in adults and neonates. With an extension to the upper genital tract, it can cause pelvic inflammatory disease and epididymitis. Disseminated gonococcal infection (DGI) is rare and characterised by petechial or pustular acral skin lesions, asymmetric polyarthralgia, tenosynovitis or oligoarticular septic arthritis [14]. Infection of the throat results from oral–genital contact and most often results in asymptomatic infection. Symptomatic infection of the oropharynx is relatively rare, but when it occurs, patients may present with multiple ulcers, a fiery red appearance of the oral mucosa with a white pseudomembrane and associated lymphadenopathy (see Chapter 13). Oral manifestations of gonorrhoea are not specific, and may mimic other conditions affecting the oropharynx including symptomatic HSV infection, erythema multiforme and immunobullous disorders [6]. Despite the fact that infection rarely causes symptoms, the oropharynx remains an important site for transmission.

Diagnosis

Diagnosis of gonorrhoea infection involves careful history taking, clinical examination and laboratory diagnostic testing. In men, urethral infection with *N. gonorrhoea* typically presents as a purulent discharge, and the demonstration of the offending organism on Gram stain of the discharge (pink diplococci within polymorphonuclear lymphocytes) provides a presumptive diagnosis, allowing immediate treatment. For penile discharge, microscopy of Gram-stained urethral smears has a sensitivity of 90–95% [23]. Microscopy of Gram-stained endocervical smears is less sensitive (30–50%) [23]. Microscopy is not used for pharyngeal specimens, as commensal species of *Neisseria* reside in the throat, which cannot be distinguished from *N. gonorrhoea* on Gram stain. NAAT is the preferred method for gonorrhoea screening using first pass urine, vaginal, cervical, rectal or throat specimens (Figure 1.4).

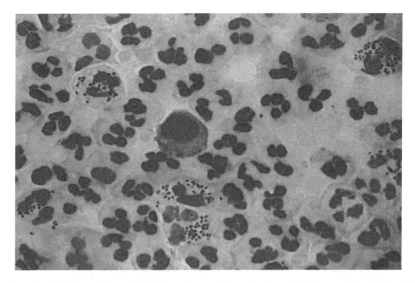

Figure 1.4 Urethral swab Gram's stain in patient with gonorrhoea [19]. Source: Joe Miller, 1979, Center for Disease Control (CDC) – PHIL/Public domain.

NAATs allow multiplex testing for chlamydial and gonococcal infections on a single specimen, and transport requirements for specimens are less stringent than for culture. To inform appropriate treatment, isolation of the organism by culture and antibiotic sensitivity testing is monitored as antimicrobial-resistant gonorrhoea is an important and emerging issue. The oropharyngeal gonococcal infections play an important role in the development of AMR in *N. gonorrhoeae* in the presence of commensal *Neisseria* species that can harbour genetic antibiotic resistance elements developed through prior antibiotic exposure [24]. Data from antimicrobial resistance testing is collected by laboratories to inform public health surveillance of this infection.

Treatment

Therapy with intramuscular *ceftriaxone 500 mg* is recommended for persons with uncomplicated gonococcal infections of the cervix, urethra, rectum or pharynx [14]. Some guidelines add 1000–2000 mg of *Azithromycin* in addition to the intramuscular *ceftriaxone* [25]. Persons who are diagnosed with gonorrhoea should be informed about the importance of contact tracing or partner notification, test of cure, when they can resume sexual activity, and STI risk reduction in future.

Viral STIs

HPV Infections

HPV infection is one of the most common STIs with approximately 40 subtypes that can potentially cause anogenital infection. The HPV types are classified based on their oncogenic potential as either low-risk (non-oncogenic) types or high-risk types (oncogenic types) (Table 1.1). Low-risk HPV types 6 and 11 cause approximately 90% of genital warts;

Table 1.1 Classification of HPV types.

Human Papillomavirus Types
Low-Risk Types (Non-Oncogenic)
- Associated with genital warts and benign or low-grade cellular changes (mild Pap test abnormalities).
- Approximately 90% of genital warts are caused by HPV types 6 and 11.
- The HPV types causing genital warts can occasionally cause lesions on oral, upper respiratory, upper gastrointestinal and ocular locations. Recurrent respiratory papillomatosis, a rare condition, is usually associated with HPV types 6 and 11.

High-Risk Types (Oncogenic)
- Associated with low-grade cervical cellular changes, high-grade cervical cellular changes (mild, moderate and severe Pap test abnormalities), and cervical dysplasia. In rare cases, associated with anogenital (i.e. cervical, vulvar, vaginal, anal and penile) and oropharyngeal cancers.
- HPV types 16 and 18 account for approximately 63% of all HPV-associated cancers and about 66% of cervical cancers.
- The HPV types 31, 33, 45, 52 and 58 cause approximately 10% of all HPV-associated cancers.

Source: Reproduced with permission from Stankiewicz Karita and Spach [26].

high-risk HPV types 16 and 18 account for approximately 63% of all HPV-associated cancers and about 70% of cervical cancers; high-risk HPV types 31, 33, 45, 52 and 58 account for an additional 10% of cervical cancers [26–28].

Epidemiology

It is estimated that most sexually active men and women will acquire genital HPV infection at some point in their lives, but most infections are asymptomatic and resolve spontaneously. Genital warts represent a sexually transmitted benign condition caused by HPV infection, especially HPV6 and HPV11. Cervical cancer is the fourth most common female malignancy [29].

Virology, Pathogenesis and Transmission

HPV is a non-enveloped, double-stranded DNA virus, approximately 50–60 nm in diameter [26]. The viral DNA genome is comprised of six early (E1, E2, E4, E5, E6 and E7) proteins that maintain regulatory function (and can cause cell oncotransformation) and two late (L1 and L2) proteins that are involved in viral assembly [30, 31]. HPV has a characteristic icosahedral viral outer shell, primarily comprised of 72 star-shaped pentameric capsomeres [30, 32]. Each pentameric capsomer contains 5 HPV L1 proteins, and each virion contains 360 of the L1 proteins [28] (Figure 1.5). All these 72 pentameric capsomers have the unique ability to self-assemble and form the outer HPV shell; this self-assembling property is the key element used in the design and production of the self-assembling HPV vaccine [33]. The viral shell also contains up to 72 molecules of the L2 minor protein, which are believed to play a role linking the capsid to the HPV DNA [28, 34].

Infection with HPV occurs at the basal cell layer of stratified squamous epithelial cells. Infection stimulates cellular proliferation in the epithelium, and the infected cells display a broad spectrum of changes that include asymptomatic infection, benign hyperplasia (papilloma), oncogenic progression and invasive carcinoma [26, 35]. To effectively replicate, HPV must utilise the host cellular machinery. During the process, the viral protein product encoded by E6 binds to the p53 tumour suppressor gene product, which results in the premature degradation of the p53 protein [36]. The E7 protein binds to a tumour suppressor protein – the retinoblastoma protein – and inhibits its function [37]. The E6 and E7 proteins mediate much of the HPV oncogenic potential by assisting the cell in evading host immunity, a process that facilitates virion production in differentiating epithelial cells [26, 28, 35].

HPV infects the mucosa of the anogenital tract, oropharyngeal region, upper respiratory tract and the surface of the skin [15]. Transmission is through skin-to-skin contact with apparent or subclinical epithelial lesions and/or through genital fluids containing infective virus during sexual activity. Resultant microabrasions enable viral inoculation and infection of the basal cells of the epithelium. Viral replication occurs in the well-differentiated layers near the surface with virions being released from desquamating cells [15].

Clinical Features

Most HPV infections are transient, asymptomatic or subclinical, and, among immunocompetent individuals, have no clinical consequences. About 90% of HPV infections are cleared by the host immune system within two years of infection. Persons with clinically evident disease have a range of possible presentations that correlate with the HPV type and host

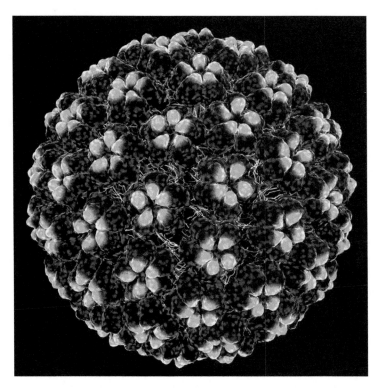

Figure 1.5 Human papillomavirus. Human papillomavirus is a small, non-enveloped, double-stranded DNA virus that is approximately 55 nm in diameter. The virus has an icosahedral shell primarily consisting of 360 molecules of the L1 major capsid protein arranged as a 72-pentameric capsomere (light blue). Source: Reproduced with permission from Stankiewicz Karita and Spach [26].

factors [26]. The most common clinically significant manifestations associated with HPV infection are anogenital warts, oral papillomas, oropharyngeal cancer, cervical cancer, cervical dysplasia, anal cancer and anal dysplasia [38, 39]. Although most precancerous lesions are not visible clinically, some will subsequently progress to form visible lesions or masses in the cervix or perianal region [26, 28].

Diseases of the oral cavity due to HPV infection include squamous papilloma, oral verrucae vulgaris, condyloma acuminatum and focal epithelial hyperplasia (Heck's disease) [6]. Squamous papilloma, associated with HPV types 6 and 11, primarily acquired through sexual activities, are the most common benign neoplasia of the oral epithelium, occurring predominantly on the soft palate, uvula and tongue. They may appear white due to keratinisation, are usually less than 1 cm in diameter, and may be fixed to the underlying tissue with a broad base (sessile) or have a stalk-like base (pedunculated) [6, 9, 40].

Verruca vulgaris, caused by HPV types 2, 4, 6 and 40 [41] are common cutaneous lesions with oral lesions affecting the keratinised tissues of the lip, hard palate and gingiva. They are solitary cauliflower-like lesions, the same colour as adjacent oral mucosa or white due to keratinisation. Transmission is often via autoinoculation of the oral or peri-oral structures from a cutaneous lesion on the finger [9].

Condyloma acuminata, caused by HPV types 6 and 11, otherwise known as genital warts, affect the anogenital epithelium but can be transmitted to the oral cavity by oral-genital contact. Oral lesions are larger than squamous papilloma and firmly adherent to underlying mucosa of the soft palate, lingual frenum and the tongue. Individual lesions coalesce to form larger lesions whose surface layer can have a cauliflower-like appearance or finger-like projections [6, 9].

Focal epithelial hyperplasia (Heck's disease) presents as small, single or multiple papules on the oral mucosa caused by infection with HPV types 13 and 32. They predominantly affect the labial and buccal mucosa, lower lip and tongue, and less commonly, the upper lip, gingiva and palate. Most lesions resolve on their own [42]. More information on HPV associated oral lesions is provided in Chapter 15.

Diagnosis

HPV types 16 and 18 are associated with approximately 70% of cervical cancers [43]. Cervical cancer screening programs rely on detecting 'high-risk' HPV types from samples of the cervix using nucleic acid hybridisation and/or cytology to identify abnormal cells and are important public health strategies employed worldwide. The oncogenic forms of HPV, types 16 and 18, are also associated with anal cancer and malignancies of the head, neck, oropharynx and oral cavity [44].

Diagnosis of HPV associated ano-genital and oral lesions relies on clinical assessment, removal and histological confirmation. Detection of a lesion during dental assessment should prompt referral with elective dental procedures being deferred until the lesion is diagnosed. The affected area should be recorded and re-examined for recurrence at each dental visit. Advising patients to stop smoking, reduce alcohol consumption and have regular dental checks is an important part of routine oral health care.

Treatment

Treatment for genital warts depends on the location of the wart. Treatments can be patient-administered (i) podophyllotoxin (Podofilox/Condylox), a derivative of podophyllin (a resin extract) with antimitotic properties and (ii) imiquimod (Aldara), a cytokine inducer that activates the cell-mediated immune system. Provider-administered treatments include (i) cryotherapy with liquid nitrogen, (ii) the caustic agents trichloroacetic acid (TCA) or bichloroacetic acid (BCA), and surgical removal [14]. Initial HPV treatments have clearance rates >50%, but recurrence is common. Treatment for cervical cancer involves chemotherapy with adjunctive radiation therapy. This type of treatment must be performed by a physician in a monitored setting due to adverse events associated with the administration of cytotoxic agents. Each cycle of chemotherapy/radiation can last multiple weeks, and patients may require several cycles to induce remission [26].

Prevention

Consistent use of latex male condoms can reduce the risk of sexual HPV transmission [14]. Vaccines can prevent diseases and cancers caused by HPV. The bivalent, quadrivalent and 9-valent HPV vaccines protect against most cervical cancer cases and the quadrivalent and 9-valent vaccines also protect against most genital warts [26]. Regular cervical cancer screenings with either pap smears or HPV DNA testing are one of the greatest preventive measures for women to lower the risk of cancer-related death. Most importantly, it is important to note that HPV vaccination does not eliminate the need for women to have regular cervical cancer screenings [26].

HSV Infections

Genital herpes is caused by both HSV type 1 (HSV1) and HSV type 2 (HSV2), but HSV2 is the most common cause of genital ulcer disease worldwide. HSV1 commonly causes oro-labial diseases (cold sores).

Epidemiology
HSV2 infection is widespread throughout the world with an estimated 491 million (13%) people aged 15–49 years worldwide living with the infection in 2016 [1].

Virology, Pathogenesis and Transmission
Both HSV1 and HSV2 are 150–200 nm α-herpesviruses that are structurally comprised of four major components: DNA, nucleocapsid, tegument and lipid envelope (Figure 1.6) [46, 47]. HSV genome is a single molecule of double-stranded DNA (approximately 152 000 base pairs that encode at least 74 genes); the DNA genome is surrounded by an icosahedral capsid, also referred to as the nucleocapsid or viral core [45]. The tegument, referred to as the matrix, is an amorphous protein-rich layer that surrounds the capsid. The envelope makes up the outermost part of HSV and consists of a lipid bilayer membrane studded with an array of 12 distinct types of glycoproteins. The glycoproteins are required for viral entry and elicit neutralising antibodies. Differences in glycoprotein G (gG) between HSV1 and HSV2 have been utilised in the development of HSV type-specific serologic tests [45].

During initial infection, HSV penetrates susceptible mucosal surfaces or abraded cracks into the skin. The virus is transported from epithelial cells to nerve endings and then along

Herpes Simplex Virus

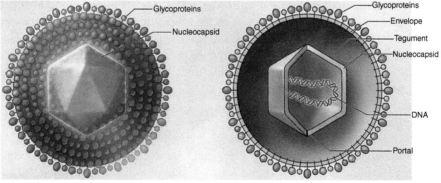

Figure 1.6 Basic structure of herpes simplex virus. Herpes simplex virus is approximately 150–200 nm in diameter. The basic structural features for HSV1 and HSV2 are the same. The image on the left depicts intact virion and that on the right shows cross-sectional view. Reproduced with permission. Source: Spach and Johnstone [45] – Illustration by Jared Travnicek, Cognition Studio.

peripheral nerve axons through retrograde transport. Once this transport is completed, HSV establishes persistent infection as an episome in the nerve cell bodies in the sacral ganglia and paraspinal ganglia [48]. In the ganglia, HSV enters a 'latent' state with an expression of viral microRNAs and the latency-associated transcript factors that are important for prevention of neuronal apoptosis, maintenance of latency and regulation of spontaneous viral reactivation [49–52]. Because HSV is not cleared from neurons, the ganglia become lifelong reservoirs for the virus [45].

Clinical Features

Traditionally, HSV2 was associated with genital disease with transmission to the genital skin through sexual contact whilst HSV1 predominantly caused oral ulceration. However, this distinction of HSV1 and HSV2 into respective sites of infection is outdated. Over the last 20 years, there has been a disproportionate rise in HSV1 as the cause of initial genital herpes infection through sexual contact in adolescence and adulthood, possibly resulting from fewer oral exposures in childhood. Conversely, HSV2 can also cause oral ulceration, although this is very uncommon compared with HSV1.

Clinical episodes of genital herpes are categorised as first-episode primary, nonprimary infection or recurrent symptomatic infection. Asymptomatic infection is common, and persons with asymptomatic or unrecognised genital herpes account for a substantial proportion of genital HSV infections [45].

Primary Genital Infection

Primary infection is defined as the first infection with either HSV1 or HSV2 in the absence of antibodies to HSV type. Primary genital infection is often symptomatic, but patients may have unrecognised or subclinical infection. With symptomatic infection, clinical manifestations of primary infection are typically more severe than recurrences and may include systemic systems and resolve within three weeks in the absence of antiviral therapy. Serum antibodies appear within 12 weeks of the primary infection in most people [45, 53, 54].

Nonprimary Infection

The term 'nonprimary HSV infection' most often refers to infection with HSV1 or HSV2 in an individual with pre-existing antibodies to the other virus. For example, a person may acquire oral HSV1 infection as a child and later acquire genital HSV2 as an adult. Manifestations of nonprimary infection tend to be milder than those of primary infection, presumably due to cross-immunity protection from prior infection with the other HSV type [45, 54, 55].

Recurrent Disease

Recurrent symptomatic genital herpes is characterised by mild, localised symptoms that typically are resolved within three to five days after onset. Prodromal symptoms (localised tingling and burning) due to HSV travelling along the nerve axons are common and begin 12–24 hours before lesions appear. Lesions typically form vesicles or pustules that progress to a wet ulcer and gradually become dry and crusted [45, 54].

Primary exposure of the oral mucosa to HSV1 (and occasionally HSV2) results in acute herpetic gingivostomatitis, typically 5–10 days after exposure to HSV. Features include fever, sore throat and painful vesicles, often in a posterior location. The characteristic vesicle of HSV breaks down to form an ulcer, scabs and eventually heals. Both keratinised and non-keratinised oral surfaces may be involved with lesions commonly located on the buccal and gingival mucosa. In severe cases, dysphagia and lymphadenopathy may be present. In immunocompetent patients, the symptoms resolve spontaneously within 10–14 days [6]. The virus migrates to the sensory ganglion in the dorsal root, innervating the primary lesion, and remains latent after initial infection [56]. Reactivation of the virus in the oral environment occurs predominantly with HSV1, causing recurrent oral disease or asymptomatic shedding. HSV2 recurrences in the oral mucosa are less common but cause more genital recurrences overall [57]. The process by which reactivation occurs is not fully understood. Potential precipitating factors include local nerve stimulation, for example by trauma or UV light, and immunosuppression secondary to other conditions such as infection or malignancy. Persistent psychological stress has also been implicated [15]. Recurrent disease presents as grouped lesions progressing from erythematous papules and vesicles to ulcerating erosions, most commonly affecting the labial tissue and vermilion [6]. Oral HSV infections are described in Chapter 14. Recurrent intraoral HSV stomatitis infection is uncommon but typically results from HSV1 infection and produces vesicles and subsequent erosions on keratinised surfaces such as the alveolar ridge, the attached gingivae, hard palate and dorsal tongue [58].

Diagnosis

The clinical diagnosis of genital HSV is challenging because many persons with genital herpes do not develop the characteristic vesicular or ulcerative lesions. Further, less typical lesions, such as fissures, can mimic other conditions. Since the natural history and subsequent clinical course depend on whether HSV1 or HSV2 is the causative agent, the clinical diagnosis of genital herpes should be confirmed by laboratory testing, including HSV typing [45, 59].

Diagnosis of genital HSV1 and HSV2 relies upon polymerase chain reaction (PCR) of viral DNA isolated from a herpetic lesion. Concentrations of HSV are much greater in the vesicle and ulcer stages, so samples from these are preferred. Serology detects previous exposure to the herpes virus and is not useful for diagnosis as up to 80% of the general population will be sero-reactive for HSV1 and about 12% for HSV2, even in the absence of clinical symptoms, due to previous exposure to the virus.

Cytologic Examination

Cells infected with HSV will show characteristic changes, and these can be observed by obtaining a sample from the lesion and smearing it on a microscope slide (e.g. Tzanck smear). This test is not recommended due to low sensitivity (less than 80%) and lack of differentiation of HSV1 from HSV2 [45].

Treatment

Oral antiviral therapy offers clinical benefits to most patients with symptomatic herpes and is the mainstay of treatment. Antiviral therapy partially controls symptoms of genital herpes when used to treat first clinical and recurrent episodes ('episodic therapy'), or when used daily to prevent recurrences or transmission ('suppressive therapy'). Antiviral therapy does not eradicate HSV, nor does it impact the risk, frequency or severity of recurrences after the medication is discontinued. Topical antiviral treatment is discouraged from clinical use since it offers less benefit than oral therapies [14]. Antiviral therapy with acyclovir, valacyclovir or famciclovir can be used intermittently for each episode of genital herpes (episodic therapy) and daily to prevent recurrent outbreaks (suppressive therapy) [45].

Dental treatment should be deferred during periods of active outbreaks of oral lesions, as retracting and stretching the skin can cause rupture of the vesicles and inoculation of the virus to adjacent skin. Aerosols or droplets created by high-speed hand pieces during procedures may contain viral particles that can infect dental staff or other areas of the patient such as the conjunctiva of the eye. Viral particles may be transmitted through tears in latex gloves, causing herpetic whitlow in the clinician. This lesion will resolve; however, dental clinicians should refrain from practice until the lesions have completely healed [9].

Prevention
Multiple strategies, including suppressive antiviral therapy, consistent use of condoms and disclosure of HSV status to partners, have been shown to reduce HSV transmission. Maximal efficacy in preventing HSV transmission is most likely achieved when a combination of these methods is used [45].

HIV Infection

HIV is a bloodborne viral pathogen that may be transmitted during unprotected sexual activity, sharing needles during injecting drug use, receiving HIV-infected organ and tissue transplants, or exposure of mucous membranes or non-intact skin with HIV-infected blood or other body fluids. HIV is a complex RNA virus of the genus *Lentivirus* within the Retroviridae family. HIV has an approximately 100 nm icosahedral structure with two single-stranded RNA molecules and 72 external spikes that are formed by the two major envelope glycoproteins, gp120 and gp41. Two major types of the HIV virus, HIV-1 and HIV-2, have been identified with HIV-1 being the most common worldwide and HIV-2 mostly found in western central Africa.

There were 37.7 million people living with HIV in 2020, up from 30.7 million in 2010, the result of continuing new infections and people living longer with HIV. Of the people living with HIV in 2020, 36 million were adults and 1.7 million were children under the age of 15 [60].

In untreated people with HIV, the disease typically progresses through three stages [61]:

Stage 1: Acute HIV infection. In this stage, infected people have a large amount of HIV in their blood. During this stage, they are highly infectious. Some people have flu-like illness with possible symptoms that may include fever, chills, rash, night sweats, muscle aches, sore throat, fatigue, swollen lymph nodes and mouth ulcers. This is the body's natural response to infection. Antigen/antibody or nucleic acid tests (NAT) are required to diagnose acute HIV infection.

Stage 2: Chronic HIV infection. This stage is also called asymptomatic HIV infection or clinical latency. HIV is still active but reproduces at lower levels. People may not have any symptoms or get sick during this phase. This period may last 5–10 years or longer. People can transmit HIV in this phase. At the end of this phase, the viral load goes up and the CD4 cell count goes down. The person may have symptoms as the virus levels increase in the body, and the person moves into Stage 3.

Stage 3: Acquired immunodeficiency syndrome (AIDS). This is the most severe phase of HIV infection. People receive an AIDS diagnosis when their CD4 cell count drops below 200 cells mm^{-1}. At this stage, opportunistic infections may manifest and can have a high degree of morbidity and even mortality.

Oral Manifestations of HIV Infection

The most common oral manifestations of HIV/AIDS include oral candidiasis, linear gingival erythema, oral hairy leukoplakia, necrotizing ulcerative gingivitis and Kaposi sarcoma. HIV/AIDS and oral lesions in HIV disease are discussed in greater detail in Chapters 5 and 11, respectively.

Sexually Acquired Viral Hepatitis

Viral hepatitis is considered an STI as hepatitis A, B and C can potentially be transmitted through sexual contact. Hepatitis B and C are potentially life-threatening liver infections and a major global health problem.

Transmission of hepatitis A virus can occur from sexual activity with an infected person mainly through faecal–oral contact. People who are sexually active are considered at risk for hepatitis A if they are MSM (men who have sex with men), live with or have sex with an infected person. Vaccination is the most effective means of preventing hepatitis A transmission among people at risk for infection [62].

Hepatitis B can be transmitted through sexual activity. Unvaccinated adults who have multiple sex partners, along with sex partners of people with chronic hepatitis B infection, are at increased risk for transmission. Most infections are acquired in childhood, but adults can acquire it through injecting–drug use with sharing of needles and syringes, and sexual contact. Hepatitis B infection acquired in adulthood leads to chronic infection in less than 5% of cases, whereas infection in infancy and early childhood leads to chronic infection in about 95% of cases. Infection with the hepatitis B virus causes hepatocellular inflammation and necrosis. Chronic infection can lead to liver fibrosis, cirrhosis and hepatocellular carcinoma (HCC). Chronic hepatitis B infection can be treated but not cured with oral antiviral agents. WHO recommends the use of oral treatments (tenofovir or entecavir) as the most potent drugs to suppress the hepatitis B virus. Most people who start hepatitis B treatment must continue it for life. Hepatitis B can be prevented by vaccines that are safe, available and effective [62, 63].

Hepatitis C virus (HCV) infection is a common cause of chronic liver disease, leading in many cases to cirrhosis, decompensated disease, liver cancer and death. It is the major cause of liver cancer and liver transplants. Although not common, hepatitis C can be transmitted through sexual activity, mainly in MSM with specific sexual and other risk factors [64]. Having an STI, having sex with multiple partners, engaging in high-risk anal sexual practices (i.e. fisting) and use of recreational drugs appear to increase the risk of acquiring hepatitis C in MSM [64]. MSM with multiple sex partners who are coinfected with HCV and HIV has been shown to be at increased risk of transmission of hepatitis C. There is no vaccine for hepatitis C. Hepatitis C has become a curable disease with the use of antiviral agents (>95%) [62].

Molluscum Contagiosum Virus Infection

Molluscum contagiosum virus (MCV) is a large DNA virus belonging to the family of poxviridae, and has four subtypes MCV1–4 [15]. MCV replicates in the cytoplasm of infected epithelial cells, presenting clinically as molluscum contagiosum with MVC1–4 being indistinguishable. Transmission occurs by direct skin-to-skin contact, which is facilitated by microabrasions and a warm, moist environment. Infectivity and extensive lesions may indicate advanced HIV infection. Diagnosis is usually made by clinical assessment, histology may show the presence of large intracytoplasmic inclusion bodies (Henderson–Patterson bodies) [65], and viral shedding occurs whilst lesions are present. Transmission can be occurred by physical contact and through fomite transmission from sharing towels. Sexual contact results in genital infection presenting as smooth, pearly, umbilicated lesions in the pubic area, thighs, buttocks and less commonly the external genitalia where it spares the mucous membranes. Autoinoculation can result in infection of the cutaneous lip and perioral skin. Lesions at these sites are flesh coloured, dome shaped, smooth or umbilicated 3–5 mm papules, often occurring in clusters [6]. They are more prevalent in the immunocompromised state.

Other STIs and Conditions

Trichomonas vaginalis (TV), a flagellated protozoan of the order Trichomonadida, is parasitic to the genitourinary tract and is the most common curable STI in the world. It does not have any oral manifestations. TV presents as a profuse malodourous vaginal discharge and vulvovaginitis in women. In 2–5% of infected women, a 'strawberry cervix' is seen on examination caused by small punctate cervical haemorrhages from the whipping motion of four anterior flagella. TV is an important diagnosis to make in pregnancy as it may be associated with premature rupture of membranes, pre-term delivery and low birth weight. TV is asymptomatic in up to 75% of men, with the most common symptom being urethral discharge. TV may be a cofactor in HIV transmission. Testing is performed using NAATs on first pass urine or high vaginal swab and/or microscopy with identification of motile protozoa propelled by flagella at 400× magnification.

Mycoplasma genitalium is a slow growing and difficult to isolate bacterium [14], preferentially colonising the urethra where it can invade epithelial cells. It is mainly transmitted by genito-genital mucosal contact with limited oral–genital transmission as oral carriage is low. It is an emerging bacterial STI, causing urethral discharge and dysuria in men and cervicitis and occasionally intermenstrual bleeding, post-coital bleeding and pelvic pain in women. Diagnosis is by NAAT on first pass urine and/or high vaginal swabs with macrolide resistance probe testing if positive to identify resistance mutations [14]. Antimicrobial resistance is a major concern in the treatment of *M. genitalium* [66] and testing and treatment may be done in consultation with a specialist.

Bacterial vaginosis (BV) is characterised by disruption of the vaginal flora with the overgrowth of anaerobic bacteria such as *Gardnerella vaginalis, Prevotella species, Mobiluncus species, Ureaplasma urealyticum and Mycoplasma hominis* replacing normally dominant *Lactobacillus* spp, thereby producing an altered vaginal discharge in women [14, 67]. BV has been implicated in PID, poor obstetric outcomes including miscarriage, preterm birth and low birth weight and increased risk of HIV acquisition [67]. Diagnosis relies on clinical features, raised vaginal pH and classical microscopic findings on Gram-stained or wet preparations of vaginal discharge.

Vulvovaginal candidiasis (VVC) is a common cause of vaginal discharge in women, and balanitis in men, most commonly due to the fungus *Candida albicans*, diagnosed by classical features of hyphae, pseudo-hyphae and spores on microscopy of a wet preparation of vaginal discharge [14]. Topical formulations of antifungal such as clotrimazole effectively treat uncomplicated VVC.

Chancroid, a rare bacterial STI, caused by the bacterium *Haemophilus ducreyi*, is characterised by painful ulceration and tender inguinal lymphadenopathy (bubo). Diagnosis relies on PCR testing of material obtained from the base of the ulcer or culture of the ulcer material [14] or pus aspirated from the bubo.

Donovanosis, another rare bacterial STI, caused by the Gram-negative bacterium *Klebsiella granulomatis*, causes chronic, slowly progressive ulceration of the genitalia. Diagnosis relies upon direct microscopy of tissue crush smear or biopsy from a lesion stained with Giemsa stain, identifying characteristic 'Donovan bodies' [14].

Scabies and pediculosis pubis (pubic lice) are genital infestations with *Sarcoptes scabiei* and *Phthirus pubis*, respectively. These are transmitted by intimate skin-to-skin contact often during sexual activity. Pubic lice are diagnosed by direct visualisation (with or without low power microscopy). Scabies is a clinical diagnosis based on the clinical finding of symmetrical polymorphic lesions on the hands (especially the finger webs), wrists, axillae, buttocks and genitals. Microscopic examination of skin scrapings allows visualisation of the mite [14].

References

1 World Health Organization (2021). Sexually transmitted infections (STIs) Fact sheet. https://www.who.int/news-room/fact-sheets/detail/ sexually-transmitted-infections-(stis).

2 Spach, D.H. and Mirchandani, M.S. (2021). Syphilis. 2e. National STD program, University of Washington, USA. Available from: https://www.std.uw.edu/go/comprehensive-study/ syphilis/core-concept/all.

3 World Health Organization (2021). Web Annex 2. Data methods. Global progress report on HIV, viral hepatitis and sexually transmitted infections, 2021 Accountability for the global health sector strategies 2016–2021: actions for impact [Internet]. Geneva: World Health Organization Licence: CC BY-NC-SA 3.0 IGO. http://apps.who.int/iris/bitstream/handle/ 10665/342813/9789240030992-eng.pdf.

4 Izard, J., Renken, C., Hsieh, C.E. et al. (2009). Cryo-electron tomography elucidates the molecular architecture of *Treponema pallidum*, the syphilis spirochete. *J. Bacteriol.* 191 (24): 7566–7580.

5 Hook, E.W. 3rd. (2017). Syphilis. *Lancet* 389 (10078): 1550–1557.

6 Bruce, A.J. and Rogers, R.S. 3rd. (2004). Oral manifestations of sexually transmitted diseases. *Clin. Dermatol.* 22 (6): 520–527.

7 Hook, E.W. III and Marra, C.M. (1992). Acquired syphilis in adults. *N. Engl. J. Med.* 326 (16): 1060–1069.

8 Ghanem, K.G., Ram, S., and Rice, P.A. (2020). The modern epidemic of syphilis. *N. Engl. J. Med.* 382 (9): 845–854.

9 NetCE (2021). Oral Manifestations of Sexually Transmitted Infections: NetCE. https://www.netce.com/coursecontent.php?courseid=1680.

10 Oswal, S. and Lyons, G. (2008). Syphilis in pregnancy. *Contin. Educ. Anaesth. Crit. Care Pain* 8 (6): 224–227.

11 Pregnancy Care Guidelines: Syphilis [22 May 2021]. Available from: www.health.gov.au/resources/pregnancy-care-guidelines/part-f-routine-maternal-health-tests/syphilis#.

12 Pessoa, L. and Galvão, V. (2011). Clinical aspects of congenital syphilis with Hutchinson's triad. *Case Rep. Dermatol.* 2011: bcr1120115130.

13 Hillson, S., Grigson, C., and Bond, S. (1998). Dental defects of congenital syphilis. *Am. J. Phys. Anthropol.* 107 (1): 25–40.

14 Workowski, K.A., Bachmann, L.H., Chan, P.A. et al. (2021). Sexually Transmitted Infections Treatment Guidelines, 2021. *MMWR Recomm. Rep.* 70 (4): 1–187.

15 Pattman, R., Sankar, N., Elawad, B. et al. (2010). *Oxford Handbook of Genitourinary Medicine, HIV, and Sexual Health.* Oxford: Oxford University Press.

16 Darville, T. and Hiltke, T.J. (2010). Pathogenesis of genital tract disease due to *Chlamydia trachomatis. J Infect Dis* 201 (Suppl 2): S114–S125.

17 David, H. and Spach, S.J. (2021).Chlamydial infections. https://www.std.uw.edu/go/comprehensive-study/chlamydial-infections/core-concept/all1

18 Öztürk, Ö. and Seven, H. (2012). *Chlamydia trachomatis* tonsillopharyngitis. *Case Rep. Otolaryngol.* 2012: 736107.

19 Spach, D. (2021). Gonococcal infection. https://www.std.uw.edu/go/comprehensive-study/gonococcal-infections/core-concept/all.

20 Cohen, M.S. and Cannon, J.G. (1999). Human experimentation with *Neisseria gonorrhoeae*: progress and goals. *J Infect Dis* 179 (Suppl 2): S375–S379.

21 Quillin, S.J. and Seifert, H.S. (2018). Neisseria gonorrhoeae host adaptation and pathogenesis. *Nat. Rev. Microbiol.* 16 (4): 226–240.

22 Hill, S.A., Masters, T.L., and Wachter, J. (2016). Gonorrhea – an evolving disease of the new millennium. *Microb. Cell.* 3 (9): 371–389.

23 Bignell, C. and FitzGerald, M. (2011). UK national guideline for the management of gonorrhoea in adults, 2011. *Int. J. STD AIDS* 22 (10): 541–547.

24 Adamson, P.C. and Klausner, J.D. (2021). The staying power of pharyngeal gonorrhea: implications for public health and antimicrobial resistance. *Clin. Infect. Dis.* 73 (4): 583–585.

25 Unemo, M., Ross, J., Serwin, A.B. et al. (2020). European guideline for the diagnosis and treatment of gonorrhoea in adults. *Int. J. STD AIDS* 2020: 956462420949126.

26 Helen C., Karita, S. and Spach, D.H. (2021). Human Papilloma virus. https://www.std.uw.edu/go/comprehensive-study/hpv/core-concept/all.

27 de Sanjose, S., Quint, W.G., Alemany, L. et al. (2010). Human papillomavirus genotype attribution in invasive cervical cancer: a retrospective cross-sectional worldwide study. *Lancet Oncol.* 11 (11): 1048–1056.

28 Schiffman, M., Doorbar, J., Wentzensen, N. et al. (2016). Carcinogenic human papillomavirus infection. *Nat. Rev. Dis. Primers.* 2: 16086.

29 Arbyn, M., Weiderpass, E., Bruni, L. et al. (2020). Estimates of incidence and mortality of cervical cancer in 2018: a worldwide analysis. *Lancet Glob. Health* 8 (2): e191–e203.

30 Doorbar, J. (2006). Molecular biology of human papillomavirus infection and cervical cancer. *Clin. Sci. (Lond.)* 110 (5): 525–541.

31 Sapp, M. and Day, P.M. (2009). Structure, attachment and entry of polyoma- and papillomaviruses. *Virology* 384 (2): 400–409.

32 Buck, C.B., Day, P.M., and Trus, B.L. (2013). The papillomavirus major capsid protein L1. *Virology* 445 (1–2): 169–174.

33 Schiller, J.T. and Davies, P. (2004). Delivering on the promise: HPV vaccines and cervical cancer. *Nat. Rev. Microbiol.* 2 (4): 343–347.

34 Wang, J.W. and Roden, R.B. (2013). L2, the minor capsid rotein of papillomavirus. *Virology* 445 (1–2): 175–186.

35 McBride, A.A. (2022). Human papillomaviruses: diversity, infection and host interactions. *Nat. Rev. Microbiol.* 20: 95–108.

36 Mantovani, F. and Banks, L. (2001). The human papillomavirus E6 protein and its contribution to malignant progression. *Oncogene* 20 (54): 7874–7887.

37 Pang, C.L. and Thierry, F. (2013). Human papillomavirus proteins as prospective therapeutic targets. *Microb. Pathog.* 58: 55–65.

38 Centers for Disease Control and Prevention (2021). Cancers Associated with Human Papillomavirus, United States—2014–2018. USCS Data Brief, no. 26. Atlanta, GA: Centers for Disease Control and Prevention, US Department of Health and Human Services.

39 Van Dyne, E.A., Henley, S.J., Saraiya, M. et al. (2018). Trends in human papillomavirus–associated cancers—United States, 1999–2015. *Morb. Mortal. Wkly. Rep.* 67 (33): 918.

40 Lynch, D.P. (2000). Oral viral infections. *Clin. Dermatol.* 18 (5): 619–628.

41 Lukes, S.M. and Meneses, M. (2010). The dental hygienist's role in HPV recognition. *Dimensions Dental Hyg.* 8 (6): 72–77.

42 Ozden, B., Gunduz, K., Gunhan, O., and Ozden, F.O. (2011). A case report of focal epithelial hyperplasia (Heck's disease) with PCR detection of human papillomavirus. *J. Maxillofacial Oral Surg.* 10 (4): 357–360.

43 Bosch, F.X., Burchell, A.N., Schiffman, M. et al. (2008). Epidemiology and natural history of human papillomavirus infections and type-specific implications in cervical neoplasia. *Vaccine* 26: K1–K16.

44 Patton, L.L. (2015). *The ADA Practical Guide to Patients with Medical Conditions.* Wiley.

45 Spach, D.H and Johnstone, C. (2021). Herpes simplex virus. https://www.std.uw.edu/go/comprehensive-study/genital-herpes/core-concept/all.

46 Kukhanova, M.K., Korovina, A.N., and Kochetkov, S.N. (2014). Human herpes simplex virus: life cycle and development of inhibitors. *Biochemistry (Mosc.)* 79 (13): 1635–1652.

47 Whitley, R.J. and Roizman, B. (2001). Herpes simplex virus infections. *Lancet* 357 (9267): 1513–1518.

48 Cunningham, A.L., Diefenbach, R.J., Miranda-Saksena, M. et al. (2006). The cycle of human herpes simplex virus infection: virus transport and immune control. *J Infect Dis* 194 (Suppl 1): S11–S18.

49 Schiffer, J.T. and Corey, L. (2013). Rapid host immune response and viral dynamics in herpes simplex virus-2 infection. *Nat. Med.* 19 (3): 280–290.

50 Perng, G.C., Jones, C., Ciacci-Zanella, J. et al. (2000). Virus-induced neuronal apoptosis blocked by the herpes simplex virus latency-associated transcript. *Science* 287 (5457): 1500–1503.

51 Umbach, J.L., Kramer, M.F., Jurak, I. et al. (2008). MicroRNAs expressed by herpes simplex virus 1 during latent infection regulate viral mRNAs. *Nature* 454 (7205): 780–783.

52 Perng, G.-C. and Jones, C. (2010). Towards an understanding of the herpes simplex virus type 1 latency-reactivation cycle. Interdiscip Perspect. *Infect. Dis.* 2010: 262415.

53 Ashley-Morrow, R., Krantz, E., and Wald, A. (2003). Time course of seroconversion by HerpeSelect ELISA after acquisition of genital herpes simplex virus type 1 (HSV-1) or HSV-2. *Sex. Transm. Dis.* 30 (4): 310–314.

54 Sawleshwarkar, S. and Dwyer, D.E. (2015). Antivirals for herpes simplex viruses. *Br. Med. J.* 351: h3350.

55 Langenberg, A.G., Corey, L., Ashley, R.L. et al. (1999). A prospective study of new infections with herpes simplex virus type 1 and type 2. Chiron HSV Vaccine Study Group. *N. Engl. J. Med.* 341 (19): 1432–1438.

56 Cook, M.L. and Stevens, J.G. (1973). Pathogenesis of herpetic neuritis and ganglionitis in mice: evidence for intra-axonal transport of infection. *Infect. Immun.* 7 (2): 272–288.

57 Scott, D., Coulter, W., and Lamey, P.J. (1997). Oral shedding of herpes simplex virus type 1: a review. *J. Oral Pathol. Med.* 26 (10): 441–447.

58 Bruce, A.J. and Rogers, R.S. (2003). Acute oral ulcers. *Dermatol. Clin.* 21 (1): 1–15.

59 Engelberg, R., Carrell, D., Krantz, E. et al. (2003). Natural history of genital herpes simplex virus type 1 infection. *Sex. Transm. Dis.* 30 (2): 174–177.

60 UNAIDS (2021). Global HIV & AIDS statistics –fact sheet, World AIDS Day https://www.unaids.org/en/resources/fact-sheet.

61 Centre for Disease Control and Prevention. About HIV/AIDS. HIV Basics. https://www.cdc.gov/hiv/basics/whatishiv.html.

62 Gilson, R. and Brook, M.G. (2006). Hepatitis A, B, and C. Sexually transmitted infections. 82 (Suppl 4): iv35–iv39.

63. World Health Organization (2021). Hepatitis B https://www.who.int/news-room/fact-sheets/detail/hepatitis-b.

64 Nijmeijer, B.M., Koopsen, J., Schinkel, J. et al. (2019). Sexually transmitted hepatitis C virus infections: current trends, and recent advances in understanding the spread in men who have sex with men. *J. Int. AIDS Soc.* 22 (Suppl 6): e25348.

65 Whitaker, S.B., Wiegand, S.E., and Budnick, S.D. (1991). Intraoral molluscum contagiosum. *Oral Surg. Oral Med. Oral Pathol.* 72 (3): 334–336.

66 Machalek, D.A., Yusha, T., Shilling, H. et al. (2020). Prevalence of mutations associated with resistance to macrolides and fluoroquinolones in *Mycoplasma genitalium* : a systematic review and meta-analysis. *Lancet Infect. Dis.* 20 (11): 1302–1314.

67 Marrazzo, J.M., Martin, D.H., Watts, D.H. et al. (2010). Bacterial vaginosis: identifying research gaps proceedings of a workshop sponsored by DHHS/NIH/NIAID. *Sex. Transm. Dis.* 37 (12): 732–744.

2

Global Epidemiology of Selected Sexually Transmitted Infections: An Overview

Yasmin Hughes[1] and Shailendra Sawleshwarkar[2]

[1]*Western Sydney Sexual Health Centre, Western Sydney Local Health District, Parramatta, New South Wales, Australia*
[2]*Sexual Health, Sydney Medical School, Faculty of Medicine and Health, University of Sydney, Sydney, Australia*

Introduction

Sexually transmitted infections (STIs) are among the most communicable conditions and a cause of physical and psychological morbidity worldwide. STIs may be caused by bacteria, viruses, protozoa, fungi or ectoparasites. In 2020, the World Health Organisation (WHO) estimated a global incidence of 374 million new cases of four curable STIs, including 128 million chlamydia cases, 82 million gonorrhoea cases, 156 million trichomoniasis cases and 7 million syphilis cases [1]. The WHO also estimated that in 2020 more than a million of people would become infected every day with one of four curable STIs: chlamydia (causative agent: *Chlamydia trachomatis*), gonorrhoea (*Neisseria gonorrhoeae*), syphilis (*Treponema pallidum*) and trichomoniasis (*Trichomonas vaginalis*) [2]. Globally, viral STIs are more common with data showing about 300 million women estimated to have human papilloma virus (HPV) infection, and more than 500 million people have genital herpes simplex virus (HSV) infection [3, 4].

The incidence, prevalence, pattern and distribution of STIs vary considerably between and within countries and regions of the world, and depend on a complex interplay of socio-economic, demographic and behavioural factors. The African region of WHO bears the largest burden of chlamydia, gonorrhoea, syphilis and trichomoniasis with 96 million incident cases followed by the Western Pacific region with 86 million. The African region has the highest prevalence of trichomoniasis in women, whereas the American region has the highest prevalence of chlamydia. The African region bears the largest burden of syphilis in both men and women.

Furthermore, each STI behaves in a unique way depending upon the biological characteristics of the causative micro-organism. The quality and extent of information on STIs also vary around the world as many resource-limited settings lack the infrastructure to make laboratory-based etiological diagnosis.

Table 2.1 Sexually transmitted infections (STIs): an overview.

STI and causative pathogen	Mode of transmission	Clinical presentations	Estimated global prevalence and incidence (WHO 2020)
Chlamydia *(Chlamydia trachomatis)*	• Sexual intercourse (vaginal, anal and oral) • Vertical • Autoinoculation (rare)	• Urethritis • Cervicitis • Proctitis • Pharyngitis • Conjunctivitis	• Prevalence: 4 and 2.5% in 15–49-year-old women and men, respectively • Incidence: 364 cases per 1000 women; 29 per 1000 men
Gonorrhoea *(Neisseria gonorrhoeae)*	• Sexual intercourse (vaginal, anal and oral) • Vertical • Autoinoculation (rare)	• Urethritis • Cervicitis • Proctitis • Pharyngitis • Conjunctivitis • Disseminated gonococcal infections and its symptoms	• Prevalence: 0.8 and 0.7% in women and men, respectively • Incidence: 19 per 1000 women and 23 per 1000 men
Syphilis *(Treponema pallidum)*	• Sexual intercourse (vaginal, anal and oral) • Vertical • Blood-borne	• Primary syphilis: anogenital and ulceration • Secondary syphilis: skin lesions, lymphadenopathy, proctitis, mucous membrane lesions, alopecia, hepatitis, meningitis, nerve deafness, iritis, anterior uveitis	• Prevalence: 0.58% in women and 0.56% in men • Incidence: 1.8 per 1000 in both women and men
Trichomonas *(Trichomonas vaginalis)*	• Sexual intercourse (vaginal)	• Urethritis (uncommon) • Cervicitis • Vulvovaginitis • Dysuria (females only) • Balanoposthitis	• Prevalence: 4.9 and 0.5% in women and men, respectively • Incidence: 38 per 1000 women and 41 per 1000 men
Herpes (4) *(Herpes simplex virus types 1 and 2)*	• Oral–oral contact • Oral–anogenital contact • Anogenital–anogenital contact	• Anogenital ulceration • Orolabial ulceration	• Prevalence of HSV2: 13.2% of global population • Incidence: 23.9 million
Genital warts (Human papilloma virus)	• Anogenital skin–skin contact	• Anogenital warts • Squamous papillomas • Oral verrucae vulgaris • Condyloma acuminatum • Focal epithelial hyperplasia • Discuss cancer here as a presentation	• Not reported

Health Consequences of STIs

Although many STIs are asymptomatic, they may have significant consequences including male and female infertility, ectopic pregnancy, cervical and other anogenital cancers. STIs cause acute urogenital syndromes such as cervicitis, urethritis, vaginitis, genital ulceration and systemic symptoms (Table 2.1). Some of these infectious agents also infect the rectum and pharynx. Another important consequence of STIs includes mother-to-child transmission, which can result in stillbirth, neonatal death, low birth weight and prematurity, sepsis, pneumonia, neonatal conjunctivitis and congenital deformities. Chlamydia and gonorrhoea are associated with chronic pelvic pain and pelvic inflammatory disease (PID) in women, leading to serious complications such as subfertility and ectopic pregnancy. Syphilis can cause neurological, cardiovascular and dermatological complications in adults. Syphilis in pregnancy is associated with stillbirth, preterm birth and congenital syphilis. Apart from the obvious ill health associated with individual STIs, there is strong evidence that STIs facilitate both the acquisition and further onward transmission of human immunodeficiency virus (HIV). STIs are also often associated with psychological distress due to the implications for intimate relationships.

Bacterial STIs are curable with antibiotic therapy. Hence, with appropriate diagnosis and treatment, bacterial STIs are potentially amenable to public health interventions. In contrast, viral STIs such as HSV and HPV infections can remain potentially infectious for prolonged periods and in the absence of symptoms. In this circumstance, without prevention of primary infection, either through behaviour modification or vaccination, the prevalence of viral STIs remains high.

Vulnerable Groups and Common Risk Factors

STIs disproportionately affect certain, vulnerable groups including young people, men who have sex with men (MSM), sex workers, people who share injecting drug equipment and people in custodial settings, further compounding health inequalities and stigma experienced by these groups. Other risk factors for STIs include multiple sexual partners, recent partner change, unprotected sexual intercourse and history of STIs. Spread of STIs in a population is determined by the rate of exposure, efficiency of transmission per exposure and duration of infectiousness, and are driven by diverse and complex set of factors for each infection.

Incidence and Prevalence of Common STIs

Syphilis

The 'syphilis epidemic' is a major health concern in many countries globally due to devastating obstetric outcomes and congenital syphilis associated with syphilis infection in pregnancy. The global prevalence for syphilis was estimated by WHO to be 0.58% in women and 0.56% in men in 2020, corresponding to a total of 22.3 million cases worldwide. The global incidence rate for syphilis was estimated as 1.8 per 1000 for men and women, translating to a total of 7.1 million syphilis cases in women and men aged 15–49 years in 2020. Africa was identified as having the highest prevalence in both males and females, whilst the Americas had the highest incidence in both sexes [1, 2]. Although overall prevalence of syphilis is 0.5% in men, prevalence in MSM across the globe remains unacceptably high. The global pooled syphilis prevalence estimate in MSM between 2000 and 2020 was 7.5% with highest pooled estimate from Latin America and the Caribbean at 10.6% and the lowest from Australia and New Zealand at 1.9% [5]. Resurgence of syphilis among MSM may be related to changes in sexual behaviour with increasing rates of new partners and concurrent partnerships, use of recreational drugs and reduced use of condoms due to pre-exposure prophylaxis for HIV [5].

Although congenital syphilis declined between 2012 and 2016, global estimates of maternal syphilis prevalence in 2016 was 0.69% resulting in a global congenital syphilis rate of 473 per 100 000 live births and 661 000 (538 000–784 000) total cases [6].

Since reaching a historic low in 2000 and 2001 in the US, rates of primary and secondary syphilis (the most infectious stages of disease) increased almost every year, increasing 11.2% during 2018–2019 among both males and females, and among all ethnic groups [7, 8]. Since 2000, rates of primary and secondary syphilis have increased among US men, likely attributable to increases among MSM who are disproportionately affected, accounting for the majority (56.7%) of cases of primary and secondary cases in 2019. Rates of primary and secondary syphilis have increased substantially in US women over recent years, increasing 30.0% during 2018–2019 and 178.6% during 2015–2019, suggesting that the heterosexual syphilis epidemic continues to increase rapidly. The 2013 rate of congenital syphilis (9.2 cases per 100 000 live births) has marked the first increase in congenital syphilis in the US since 2008 with the rate increasing year on year since then with 1870 cases as reported in 2019 [9].

In 2018, about 33 927 confirmed syphilis cases were reported in 29 EU countries, giving a crude notification rate of 7.0 cases per 100 000 population with increasing trend since 2011 up to 2017, particularly among MSM [10]. For the first time, since 2013, the number of notified cases of congenital syphilis has increased in 2018 with 60 reported in 23 EU countries, a crude rate of 1.6 cases per 100 000 live births [11]. Syphilitic infection and congenital syphilis remain public health priorities in the UK. There was about 10% increase in syphilis (primary, secondary and early latent stages) between 2018 and 2019 with notable increases in both heterosexual women and men. Although the increase in MSM was minimal, the MSM population bears the largest burden of syphilis. Nine cases of congenital syphilis were reported in England in 2019 highlighting the importance of screening and treatment of this infection in pregnancy [12].

In Australia, infectious syphilis notifications have increased since 2010 in both men and women, particularly in women aged 15–44 years [5]. Between 2013 and 2017, the notification rate of infectious syphilis increased by 135%, from 7.8 per 100 000 in 2013 to 18.3 per 100 000 in 2017, with an increase in both men (119%) and women (309%) [13]. The rate of notification for infectious syphilis among Aboriginal and Torres Strait Islander women was 40 times greater than among non-indigenous women [14]. Coinciding with peaks in infectious syphilis notifications, there have been peaks in cases of congenital syphilis. Between 2008 and 2017, 59% of the 44 congenital syphilis notifications were in the Aboriginal and Torres Strait Islander population [14]. Targeted syphilis screening and diagnosis in pregnancy remain a public health priority in both high-income and low-income settings worldwide

Chlamydia

Chlamydia remains the most commonly diagnosed bacterial STIs in high-income countries despite widespread testing recommendations, sensitive and specific non-invasive testing, and cheap and effective therapy [15]. A large proportion of genital chlamydia infections are asymptomatic. Sexually active young individuals are most at risk of chlamydia, and women aged 15–29 years have the highest number of infections worldwide.

Chlamydial infections are a major public health issue, because of the asymptomatic nature of most infections allowing for onward transmission and the long-term complications that can arise from undiagnosed infections especially in women such as PID and tubal damage with risk of ectopic pregnancy and infertility. Since the potential for significant morbidity with chlamydia infection, screening and treatment in young women remains public health priorities.

Globally, there were a total of 128.5 million cases of chlamydia in 2020 with prevalence values of 4.0 and 2.5% in 15–49-year-old women and men, respectively. Compared with 2016, the prevalence has increased in women from 3.8 to 4.0% and declined in men from 2.7 to 2.5%. Prevalence was highest in the Americas for women and in Africa for men. The global incidence rate for chlamydia was estimated as 36 cases per 1000 women and 29 per 1000 men in 2020, translating to 128.5 million new chlamydia cases with the highest incidence rate for both men and women being in the Americas [1, 16].

In 2019, the Centre for Disease Control and Prevention (CDC) reported a total of 1.8 million cases of *C. trachomatis*, making it the most common notifiable condition in the US that year and a 2.8% increased rate of infection compared to the previous year [8, 9]. Increases were reported in both males and females and in all ethnic groups. Rates of reported chlamydia were highest among adolescents and young adults: in 2019, almost two-third cases (61%) were among persons aged 15–24 years [9].

Similar trends have been reported by Public Health England, UK. In 2019, the most commonly diagnosed STI was chlamydia, accounting for 49% of all new STI diagnoses. Compared to 2018, there was a 5% increase in chlamydia cases diagnosed. Between 2018 and 2019, chlamydia diagnoses remained stable among heterosexual women and decreased slightly among heterosexual men (2%) but increased sharply in women who have sex with women (WSW) (79%) and, to a lesser extent, in MSM (21%) [12]. In 2018, 26 countries in EU reported 406 406 confirmed chlamydia infections with crude notification rate of 146 per 100 000 population with a stable but high notification rate over the last five years [17]. The UK accounted for 60% of all reported cases in the EU.

Chlamydia notification rates in Australia were slightly reduced in 2019 from 2018 overall (423.2 per 100 000 compared to 429.5 per 100 000) and in men (409.4 per 100 000 compared to 410 per 100 000) and women (439.8 per 100 000 compared to 451.7 per 100 000) [13].

Gonorrhoea

Globally, WHO estimated the prevalence of gonorrhoea to be 0.9% in women and 0.7% in men with a total of 30.6 million cases in 2016. The highest prevalence and incidence of gonorrhoea in both men and women were estimated to lie in Africa. The global incidence rate for gonorrhoea was estimated to be 20 per 1000 women and 26 per 1000 men, translating into 86.9 million cases of gonorrhoea in women and men aged 15–49 years in 2016 [1, 2].

Gonorrhoea has been highlighted by the CDC as a public health priority due to the growing concern of antimicrobial resistance (AMR) and multidrug-resistant gonorrhoea. In 2019, a total of 616 392 cases of gonorrhoea were reported to the CDC, making it the second most common notifiable condition in the US for that year. There was a 5.5% increase in the overall rate of gonorrhoea during 2018–2019 with increases reported in both men, women, and in all racial and ethnic groups. Since 2013, gonorrhoea has been higher in men compared to women in the US, and this trend continued from 2018 to 2019 with rates increasing in both groups but larger increases seen in men (43.6% increase in women and 60.6% increase in men in 2015–2019). Data from the STD Surveillance Network suggests that estimated rates of reported gonorrhoea among MSM are 42 times the estimated rate among men who have sex with women, although reported rates in MSM have slowed down in the last several years [9].

A total of 100,673 confirmed cases of gonorrhoea were reported by 28 EU member states for 2018 with an overall crude notification rate of 26.4 cases per 100 000 population. MSM accounted for almost half of the reported cases [18]. Rates of reported gonorrhoea infections continued to increase in the majority of EU over the last decade, driven largely by increased notifications in MSM as well as women [18]. Like the US, gonorrhoea was the second most common STI diagnosed in England in 2019 (15% of all diagnoses) and had the largest increase in infections compared to 2018 of all STIs (26%; from 56 232 to 70 936). The number of gonorrhoea diagnoses in 2019 was the largest annual number reported since records began in 1918 and is a continuation of the increasing trend seen in recent years. Since 2015, gonorrhoea diagnoses have risen by 71% (from 41 382 to 70 936). While the majority of gonorrhoea diagnoses were reported in MSM over the same period, diagnoses have also increased notably in women and heterosexual men. Between 2018 and 2019, increases in gonorrhoea were reported in all age groups of people aged 15 years and older, with the largest proportional increase in people aged 20–24 years (28%; from 13 623 to 17 443). [12]

Similarly, notifications of gonorrhoea have steadily increased during 2010–2019 in Australia, especially in men. From 2018 to 2019 alone, gonorrhoea cases increased from 186.0 per 100 000 to 200.9 per 100 000 in men and 67.6 per 100 000 to 76.8 per 100 000 in women. [13, 19]

Another critical aspect of gonococcal infections is AMR and rapidly changing antimicrobial susceptibility. WHO runs the Global Gonococcal Antimicrobial Surveillance Programme (GASP) to identify and monitor AMR and to inform updates to the treatment guidelines. Gonococcal resistance is very common to penicillin, tetracycline and to quinolones. Recently, increasing gonococcal resistance has been reported with oral extended spectrum cephalosporin, and clinical treatment failure with the injectable cephalosporin, ceftriaxone, has occasionally been reported, raising concerns about the spread of extensively drug-resistant gonococcal infections [20].

Trichomoniasis

Trichomoniasis is a sexually transmitted vaginitis caused by the single-celled protozoan parasite *T. vaginalis* and is the most common curable STI globally with a total of

156 million cases reported in 2020. WHO estimated the global pooled prevalence to be 4.9% in women and 0.5% in men in 2020 with the region of Africa and the Americas having the highest prevalence for women and men, respectively. The global incidence of trichomoniasis among 15–49 years old was estimated as 38 per 1000 women and 41 per 1000 men in 2020, with African and American regions being identified as having the highest incidence in both men and women [1, 2]. Whilst common in low-income settings, trichomoniasis is relatively uncommon in high-income countries such as the US, the UK and Australia, where it disproportionately affects certain populations.

In the US from 2013 to 2016, the prevalence of *T. vaginalis* was reported as 2.1% among women and 0.5% among men aged 14–59, based on a nationally representative sample [21]. For both men and women, poverty, lower educational level, unmarried status and having been born in the US were associated with *T. vaginalis* infection in this study. For women, younger age at first intercourse, greater number of sex partners and a history of chlamydia infection in the past 12 months were associated with *T. vaginalis* infection [21].

T. vaginalis is uncommon in the UK [22]. Studies have reported that *T. vaginalis* in England is more common in those from ethnic minority populations [22, 23]. In Australia, the reported prevalence of trichomoniasis varies in different regions, with no cases in urban areas [24, 25] and increasing cases in regional and remote communities [24]. Risk factors include multiple sexual partners, previous STI(s), sex work, intravenous drug use, low socioeconomic status and incarceration [25, 26].

Human Papilloma Virus

HPV is the most common viral infection of the reproductive tract and has gained much attention due to the role of certain 'high-risk oncogenic types' in the development of cervical, anal and oropharyngeal cancers. Cervical cancer is the eighth most common cancer globally, with approximately 570 000 women diagnosed with cervical cancer and 311 000 deaths every year. The majority of cases occur in low-income countries where there are no formal, freely accessible prevention or screening programmes [27, 28]. Whilst there are over 100 strains of HPV, and infection with HPV is very common across the population, two strains (HPV 16 and 18) account for over 70% of cervical cancers [29]. Cervical cancer accounts for 83% of HPV-attributable cancers, two-thirds of which occur in less-developed countries [30]. Genital warts are caused by low-risk HPV types 6 and 11 in more than 90% of cases and are a common cause for attendance to sexual health clinics. It is estimated that most sexually active men and women will acquire HPV infection at some point, but most will remain asymptomatic, with the infection clearing spontaneously. As genital warts are not in a reportable condition in many countries, the true prevalence and incidence of this condition are unknown.

There is good evidence for the carcinogenic role of HPV type 16 in oral and oropharyngeal cancers. Around 30% of oropharyngeal cancers (which mainly comprises the tonsils and base of tongue sites) are caused by HPV with HPV16 being the most frequent type [28, 30].

The introduction of the quadrivalent and the more recent nonavalent HPV vaccine (which protect against HPV types 6 and 11 in addition to oncogenic types) has led to marked reductions in genital warts and HPV infections in young women and men in many countries [31]. Public Health England reported substantial reductions in genital wart diagnoses in young women, the majority of whom were vaccinated. They also reported declines in similar-aged heterosexual unvaccinated young men that are likely attributable to substantial herd immunity [12]. Australian data have also shown significant and ongoing reduction in genital warts in both Australian-born female individuals and heterosexual male individuals after the introduction of the national HPV vaccination program with less than 1% diagnosed with genital warts in 15- to 20-year-old age groups since 2015 [32].

Herpes Simplex Virus

Genital herpes is the leading cause of genital ulcer disease worldwide. Although both herpes simplex virus type 1 (HSV1) and herpes simplex virus type 2 (HSV2) can potentially cause genital ulceration, most cases worldwide are seen with HSV2 infection. HSV1 is primarily transmitted by oral–oral contact and mostly causes orolabial symptoms [33]. Most infections with HSV1 are acquired in childhood. HSV1 and HSV2 infections are lifelong. In 2016, an estimated 3.7 billion people under the age of 50 or 67% of the population, had HSV1 infection (oral or genital). Most genital HSV1 infections are estimated to occur in the Americas, Europe and Western Pacific where HSV1 infection may occur less frequently during childhood, leaving adolescents, young adults, and adults, vulnerable to this infection and with potential to acquire it during sex [4].

HSV2 infection is widespread with an estimated 491 million (13%) people aged 15–49 years worldwide living with the infection in 2016 [4]. More women are estimated to be infected with HSV2 than men (313 million women and 178 million men in 2016) likely due to the easier transmission of infection from men to women. Prevalence of HSV2 infection was estimated to be highest in Africa followed by the Americas [4].

HIV/AIDS

According to WHO, there were an estimated number of 37.7 million (30.2–45.1 million) people living with HIV at the end of 2020, over two thirds of whom (25.4 million) are in the WHO African Region. In 2020, 1.5 million people acquired HIV [2]. Regional data of the infection has been presented in Chapter 5.

Summary

Over the last few decades, continuing advances in diagnostics and therapeutics as well as better data collection across the world have provided better understanding of the epidemiology of STIs. This has led to evidence-based public health interventions and health promotion approaches to minimise the impact of STIs on individuals and populations. Despite the progress in control of STIs, incidence of most STIs has plateaued. More than 1 million curable STIs are acquired every day worldwide, caused by *C. trachomatis, N. gonorrhoeae, T. pallidum (syphilis) and T. vaginalis*. Additionally, about 500 million people have genital herpes, and the burden of HPV-related diseases remains high in developing countries.

Recent increases in bacterial STIs warrant urgent attention while HPV vaccination efforts require strengthening in low- and middle-income countries. With increasing use of pre-exposure prophylaxis for HIV prevention, it is important to pay more attention to the changing epidemiologic parameters for STIs to better target public health interventions for STI control and prevention.

References

1 World Health Organization (2021). Sexually transmitted infections (STIs) Fact sheet. https://ww w.who.int/news-room/fact-sheets/detail/sexually-transmitted-infections-(stis).

2 World Health Organization (2021). Web Annex 2. Data methods. Global progress report on HIV, viral hepatitis, and sexually transmitted infections, 2021 Accountability for the global health sector strategies 2016–2021: actions for impact [Internet]. Geneva: World Health Organization. Licence: CC BY-NC-SA 3.0 IGO. http://apps.who.int/iris/bitstream/handle/10665/342813/9789240030992-eng.pdf.

3 de Sanjosé, S., Diaz, M., Castellsagué, X. et al. (2007). Worldwide prevalence, and genotype distribution of cervical human papillomavirus DNA in women with normal cytology: a meta-analysis. *Lancet Infect. Dis.* 7 (7): 453–459.

4 James, C., Harfouche, M., Welton, N.J. et al. (2020). Herpes simplex virus: global infection prevalence and incidence estimates, 2016. *Bull. World Health Organ.* 98 (5): 315–329.

5 Tsuboi, M., Evans, J., Davies, E.P. et al. (2021). Prevalence of syphilis among men who have sex with men: a global systematic review and meta-analysis from 2000–2013;20. *Lancet Global Health* 9 (8): e1110–e1118.

6 Korenromp, E.L., Rowley, J., Alonso, M. et al. (2019). Global burden of maternal and congenital syphilis and associated adverse birth outcomes – estimates for 2016 and progress since 2012. *PLoS One* 14 (2): e0211720.

7 Centers for Disease Control and Prevention (2021). *Syphilis Surveillance Supplemental Slides, 2015–2019*. Atlanta: U.S. Department of Health and Human Services.

8 Centers for Disease Control and Prevention (2019). Sexually Transmitted Disease Surveillance 2019 Atlanta: U.S. Department of Health and Human Services. https://www .cdc.gov/std/statistics/2019/default.htm

9 Centers for Disease Control and Prevention (2019). National Overview-Sexually Transmitted Disease Surveillance. https://www.cdc.gov/std/statistics/2019/overview.htm#Chlamydia.

10 European Centre for Disease Prevention and Control (2020). Syphilis. ECDC. Annual epidemiological report for 2018 Stockholm: ECDC

11 European Centre for Disease Prevention and Control (2020). Congenital syphilis. ECDC. Annual epidemiological report for 2018. Stockholm: ECDC.

12 Ratna, N.S.T., Glancy, M., Sun, S. et al. (2020). MHac. Sexually transmitted infections and screening for chlamydia in England. London: Public Health England; 2021.

13 National update on HIV, viral hepatitis and sexually transmissible infections in Australia: 2009–2018 (2020). Sydney: Kirby Institute, UNSW Sydney.

14 Aboriginal Surveillance Report on HIV, viral hepatitis and STIs 2018 Sydney: Kirby Institute, UNSW (2021). https://kirby.unsw.edu.au/report/Aboriginal- surveillance-report-hiv-viral-hepatitis-and-stis-2018.

15 Unemo, M., Bradshaw, C.S., Hocking, J.S. et al. (2017). Sexually transmitted infections: challenges ahead. *Lancet Infect. Dis.* 17 (8): e235–e279.

16 Rowley, J., Vander Hoorn, S., Korenromp, E. et al. (2019). Chlamydia, gonorrhoea, trichomoniasis and syphilis: global prevalence and incidence estimates, 2016. *Bull. World Health Organ.* 97 (8): 548–62P.

17 European Centre for Disease Prevention and Control (2020). Chlamydia infection. ECDC. Annual epidemiological report for 2018. Stockholm: ECDC.

18 European Centre for Disease Prevention and Control (2020). Gonorrhoea. ECDC. Annual epidemiological report for 2018. Stockholm: ECDC.

19 Sexually transmissible infections Sydney (2021). Kirby Institute, UNSW https://data.kirby .unsw.edu.au/STIs.

20 Wi, T., Lahra, M.M., Ndowa, F. et al. (2017). Antimicrobial resistance in *Neisseria gonorrhoeae*: global surveillance and a call for international collaborative action. *PLoS Med.* 14 (7): e1002344.

21 Flagg, E.W., Meites, E., Phillips, C. et al. (2019). Prevalence of *Trichomonas vaginalis* among civilian, noninstitutionalized male and female population aged 14 to 59 years: United States, 2013 to 2016. *Sex Transm. Dis.* 46 (10): e93–e96.

22 Field, N., Clifton, S., Alexander, S. et al. (2018). *Trichomonas vaginalis* infection is uncommon in the British general population: implications for clinical testing and public health screening. *Sex. Transm. Infect.* 94 (3): 226.

23 Mitchell, H.D., Lewis, D.A., Marsh, K., and Hughes, G. (2014). Distribution and risk factors of *Trichomonas vaginalis* infection in England: an epidemiological study using electronic health records from sexually transmitted infection clinics, 2009–2011. *Epidemiol Infect.* 142 (8): 1678–1687.

24 Ryder, N., Woods, H., McKay, K. et al. (2012). *Trichomonas vaginalis* prevalence increases with remoteness in rural and remote New South Wales, Australia. *Sex Transm. Dis.* 39 (12): 938–941.

25 Johnston, V.J. and Mabey, D.C. (2008). Global epidemiology and control of *Trichomonas vaginalis*. *Curr. Opin. Infect. Dis.* 21 (1): 56–64.

26 Brown, D. Jr. (2004). Clinical variability of bacterial vaginosis and trichomoniasis. *J. Reprod. Med.* 49 (10): 781–786.

27 Arbyn, M., Weiderpass, E., Bruni, L. et al. (2020). Estimates of incidence and mortality of cervical cancer in 2018: a worldwide analysis. *Lancet Glob. Health* 8 (2): e191–e203.

28 Bruni, L.A.G., Serrano, B., Mena, M. et al. (2021). Human Papillomavirus and Related Diseases in the World. Summary Report 22 October 2021. ICO/IARC Information Centre on HPV and Cancer (HPV Information Centre).

29 de Sanjose, S., Quint, W.G., Alemany, L. et al. (2010). Human papillomavirus genotype attribution in invasive cervical cancer: a retrospective cross-sectional worldwide study. *Lancet Oncol.* 11 (11): 1048–1056.

30 de Martel, C., Plummer, M., Vignat, J., and Franceschi, S. (2017). Worldwide burden of cancer attributable to HPV by site, country and HPV type. *Int. J. Cancer* 141 (4): 664–670.

31 Drolet, M., Bénard, É., Pérez, N. et al. (2019). Population-level impact and herd effects following the introduction of human papilloma virus vaccination programmes: updated systematic review and meta-analysis. *Lancet* 394 (10197): 497–509.

32 Chow, E.P.F., Carter, A., Vickers, T. et al. (2021). Effect on genital warts in Australian female and heterosexual male individuals after introduction of the national human papillomavirus gender-neutral vaccination programme: an analysis of national sentinel surveillance data from 2004–2013;18. *Lancet Infect. Dis.* 21 (12): 1747–1756.

33 Higgins, C.R., Schofield, J.K., Tatnall, F.M., and Leigh, I.M. (1993). Natural history, management and complications of herpes labialis. *J. Med. Virol.* (Suppl 1): 22–26.

3

Impact of Sexually Transmitted Diseases on Public Health

Chythra R. Rao[1] and Raghavendra Rao[2]

[1]Department of Community Medicine, Kasturba Medical College, Manipal, India
[2]Department of Dermatology, Kasturba Medical College, Manipal, India

Introduction

Sexually transmitted infections (STIs) pose major health and economic challenges globally. More than 1 million STIs are acquired every day worldwide [1]. STIs are one of the leading causes of morbidity and mortality, as measured by disability-adjusted life years (DALYs) for reproductive-aged women [2]. For all sexually transmitted diseases (STDs), a major problem for society is the amount of money spent on the screening, diagnosis and treatment of infections.

Although multiple bacterial and viral agents have been incriminated for various STIs, behavioural risk factors, low socio-economic status, migration, and lack of awareness continue to drive the ongoing epidemic of STIs, as outlined in Figure 3.1. In the low- and middle-income countries, the high levels of STIs are largely due to delayed or inadequate diagnosis and treatment of STIs, inadequacies in health service provision and healthcare seeking [3]. Recent data reported from high-income countries suggest a trend towards initiation of sex at a younger age, greater frequency of same sex and bisexual behaviours, and greater frequency of oral and anal sex risky behaviours, particularly among younger cohorts that include large numbers of sex partners, indiscriminate choice of sex partners, short periods between the time two people meet each other and the initiation of sexual activity, short time spent during the sexual encounter, lack or short duration of social links between sex partners, short duration of gaps between consecutive sex partners and sexual encounters, and a tendency for both partners to recruit each other for sex [4].

STIs are spread predominantly by sexual contact, including vaginal, anal and oral sex. Some STIs can also be transmitted from mother to child during pregnancy, childbirth and breastfeeding [1, 5].

Sexually Transmissible Oral Diseases, First Edition.
Edited by S.R. Prabhu, Nicholas van Wagoner, Jeff Hill and Shailendra Sawleshwarkar.
© 2023 John Wiley & Sons Ltd. Published 2023 by John Wiley & Sons Ltd.

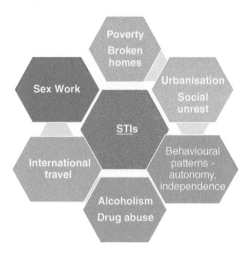

Figure 3.1 Behavioural and social determinants of STIs.

Impact on General and Sexual Health

STIs demonstrate an iceberg phenomenon. Most of the patients may be asymptomatic. Common symptoms of STIs include vaginal discharge, urethral discharge or burning in men, genital ulcers and abdominal pain. Even when symptomatic, health-seeking behaviour may be poor because of stigma, lack of awareness, self-medication and belief in traditional systems of medicine.

STIs have direct impact on sexual and reproductive health through stigmatisation, infertility, cancers and pregnancy complications. STIs like herpes, gonorrhoea and syphilis can increase the risk of acquiring human immunodeficiency virus (HIV). Transmission of STIs from mother to child can result in stillbirth, neonatal death, low-birth weight and prematurity, sepsis, pneumonia, neonatal conjunctivitis and congenital deformities [1].

Hepatitis B resulted in an estimated 820 000 deaths in 2019, mostly from cirrhosis and hepatocellular carcinoma (primary liver cancer). Human papillomavirus (HPV) infection causes cervical cancer. Cervical cancer is the fourth most common cancer among women globally, with an estimated 570 000 new cases in 2018 and over 311 000 cervical cancer deaths every year [6]. Gonococcal infections represent 106 million new cases of curable STIs that occur globally every year. The emergence of drug resistance to cephalosporins in *Neisseria gonorrhoeae*, together with the longstanding resistance to penicillins, sulfonamides, tetracyclines and, more recently, quinolones and macrolides (including azithromycin), is a cause for concern [7].

Prevention Challenges

A comprehensive people-centric primary-care-driven, equitable, accessible, affordable health system with intersectoral co-ordination and adequate community participation is needed to adequately address the burden of STIs. The modes of intervention at various levels of prevention strategies are summarised in Figure 3.2.

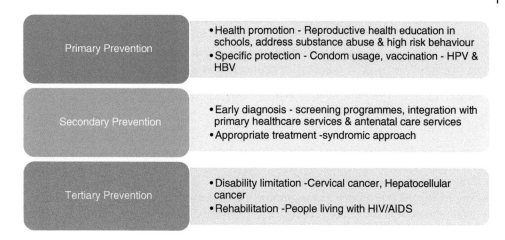

Figure 3.2 Summary of prevention strategies for control of STIs.

Family Health Awareness Campaign (FHAC) launched in 1999, by the National AIDS Control Organization (NACO), Ministry of Health, and Government of India, aims at creating awareness in the community regarding respiratory tract infections (RTI)/STD/HIV–acquired immunodeficiency syndrome (AIDS) through home visits and village-based camps and encouraging clients suspected to have RTI/STD to seek early treatment [8]. South Africa has launched a multidisease national wellness campaign to accelerate screening and testing for HIV, tuberculosis, STIs and non-communicable diseases, including hypertension and diabetes [9]. Such approaches are effective in controlling the spread of STIs.

Diagnostic and Management Challenges

Diagnostic tests for STIs are expensive and not easily available, and affordable for most of the population in low- and middle-income countries. The only inexpensive, rapid tests currently available for STIs are for syphilis, hepatitis B and HIV. These are being scaled up to ensure that all pregnant women are offered these tests at the first antenatal care visit. Elimination of mother-to-child transmission of HIV, syphilis and hepatitis B – 'triple elimination initiative', promoted by the World Health Organization (WHO), includes testing for HIV, syphilis and HBV in antenatal care clinics, counselling, treatment and appropriate care and follow-up of the child [10]. Effective treatment is currently available for several STIs. Chlamydia, gonorrhoea, syphilis and trichomoniasis are generally curable with existing single-dose regimens of antibiotics. For herpes and HIV, antivirals are available to modulate the course of the disease, but do not offer cure. For hepatitis B, antiviral medications slow the damage to the liver, but are expensive and not easily available. WHO has recommended syndromic management using easily recognisable signs and symptoms to guide treatment, without the use of laboratory tests. Low- and middle-income countries rely on these clinical algorithms, which allow even health workers to diagnose specific infections (e.g. vaginal discharge, urethral discharge, genital ulcers and abdominal pain) [11, 12]. Syndromic management is simple, assures rapid, same-day treatment and avoids expensive or unavailable diagnostic tests for patients that present with symptoms. In order to interrupt transmission of infection and prevent re-infection, treating sexual partners is an important component of STI case management [13].

Challenges in Control of STIs

Challenges to control of STIs are numerous [14]. These can be listed as follows:

- Low priority in resource allocation
- Identifying the true burden and controlling the spread of disease
- Failure to address the socio-behavioural risk factors, illiteracy, unemployment and sub-stance abuse
- Initiating and sustaining behaviour change to address high-risk behaviour
- Challenges in partner notification and contact tracing
- Lack of public awareness, lack of training among health workers, and stigma around STIs
- Limited resources, lack of access to health services for screening and treatment, poor quality of services and out-of-pocket expenses
- Lack of funding for screening, limited laboratory capacity and inadequate supplies of appropriate medicines

The effective prevention and care of STDs can be achieved using a combination of responses, including the 'public health package'. STD service delivery should be expanded to embrace the public health package. Some of the components of the public health package are discussed in more detail in the following sections.

In 1998, United Nations Program on HIV/AIDS (UNAIDS) outlined in the public health package for STI prevention and care components of which are outlined in Box 3.1 [15].

Box 3.1   The Public Health Package for STD Prevention and Care: The Essential Components

- Promotion of safer sex behaviour
- Condom programming – encompassing a full range of activities from condom promotion to the planning and management of supplies and distribution .
- Promotion of healthcare-seeking behaviour
- Integration of STD control into primary healthcare, reproductive healthcare facilities, private clinics and others.
- Specific services for populations with often high-risk behaviours – such as female and male sex workers, adolescents, long-distance truck drivers, military personnel and prisoners
- Comprehensive case management of STDs
- Prevention and care of congenital syphilis and neonatal conjunctivitis
- Early detection of symptomatic and asymptomatic infections

Source: UNAIDS [15].

Global Health Sector Strategy on Ending STIs

WHO strongly advocates the need for the global health sector strategy towards ending STIs [16]. The strategy outlines how to ensure equitable coverage of services and maximum impact for all people in need, which focusses on both the general population and specific population groups.

The components of the strategy include the following:

- Each country needs to define the specific populations that are most affected by STI epidemics.
- The response should be based on the epidemiological as well as social context.
- Specific populations that focus on STIs will include populations most likely to have a high number of sex partners, such as sex workers and their clients.
- Other populations for consideration include men who have sex with men, transgendered people and people with an existing STI, including people living with HIV. Most of these groups overlap with groups recognised as key populations for HIV.
- Other groups, considered to be particularly vulnerable to STIs, include young people and adolescents, women, mobile populations, children and young people living on the street, prisoners, drug users and people affected by conflict and civil unrest.

References

1 World Health Organization (2021). Sexually Transmitted Diseases. https://www.who.int/news-room/fact-sheets/detail/sexually-transmitted-infections-(stis). (Accessed on Jan 8th, 2022)

2 Kamb, M.L., Lackritz, E., Mark, J. et al. (2007). Sexually Transmitted Infections in Developing Countries: Current Concepts and Strategies on Improving STI Prevention, Treatment, and Control. Working Paper 42797, World Bank, Washington, DC

3 Aral, S.O., Hogben, M., and Wasserheit, J.N. (2008). STD-related health care seeking and health service delivery. In: *Sexually Transmitted Diseases* (ed. K.K. Holmes, P.F. Sparling, W.E. Stamm, et al.). New York: McGraw-Hill.

4 Aral, S.O. and Ward, H. (2014). Behavioral convergence: implications for mathematical models of sexually transmitted infection transmission. *J. Infect. Dis.* 210 (Suppl 2): S600–S604.

5 Chesson, H.W., Mayaud, P., and Aral, S.O. (2017). Sexually transmitted infections: impact and cost-effectiveness of prevention. In: *Major Infectious Diseases*, 3e (ed. K.K. Holmes, S. Bertozzi, B.R. Bloom, et al.). Washington (DC): The International Bank for Reconstruction and Development/The World Bank Chapter 10. https://www.ncbi.nlm.nih.gov/books/NBK525195. http://dx.doi.org/10.1596/978-1-4648-0524-0_ch10.

6 Bray, F., Ferlay, J., Soerjomataram, I. et al. (2018). Global cancer statistics 2018: GLOBOCAN estimates of incidence and mortality worldwide for 36 cancers in 185 countries. *CA Cancer J. Clin.* 68 (6): 394–424. https://doi.org/10.3322/caac.21492. Epub 2018 Sep 12. Erratum in: (2020). CA Cancer J. Clin. 70(4): 313. https://doi.org/10.1371/journal.pone.0211720.

7 Global action plan to control the spread and impact of antimicrobial resistance in *Neisseria gonorrhoeae*. http://apps.who.int/iris/bitstream/handle/10665/44863/9789241503501_eng .pdf?sequence=1 (Accessed on Jan 10th 2022)

8 Family health awareness campaigns in India. http://inclentrust.org/inclen/wp-content/ uploads/2015/02/42.-Family-Health-Awareness-concurrent-evaluation.pdf (Accessed on Feb 20th 2022)

9 Cheka Impilo campaign in Africa. https://sanac.org.za/the-national-wellness-campaign-cheka-impilo (Accessed on Feb 25th 2022)

10 Elimination of mother-to-child transmission of HIV, syphilis and hepatitis B. https://www .who.int/initiatives/triple-elimination-initiative-of-mother-to-child-transmission-of-hiv-syphilis-and-hepatitis-b (Accessed on Feb 20th 2022)

11 Guidelines for the management of sexually transmitted infections. https://www.who.int/ hiv/topics/vct/sw_toolkit/guidelines_management_sti.pdf (Accessed on Feb 20th 2022)

12 Guidelines for the management of symptomatic sexually transmitted infections. https:// www.who.int/publications/i/item/9789240024168 (Accessed on Feb 20th 2022)

13 Syndromic management for STI. www.naco.gov.in/sites/default/files/Medical%20 Officer%20Handout.pdf (accessed on Feb 20th, 2022)

14 Mayaud, P. and Mabey, D. (2004). Approaches to the control of sexually transmitted infections in developing countries: old problems and modern challenges. *Sex. Transm. Infect.* 80: 174–182.

15 UNAIDS (1998). The public health approach to STD control: UNAIDS Technical Update. UNAIDS Best Practice Collection: Technical Update Geneva: UNAIDS.

16 Global health sector strategy on Sexually Transmitted Infections, 2016–2021. (2016). https://www.who.int/publications/i/item/WHO-RHR-16.09 (Accessed on Jan 8th, 2022)

4

Sexually Transmitted Infection Prevention: An Overview

S.R. Prabhu[1], Amanda Oakley[2] and David H. Felix[3]

[1]University of Queensland, School of Dentistry, Brisbane, Australia
[2]Department of Medicine, University of Auckland, New Zealand
[3]NHS Education for Scotland, Edinburgh and School of Medicine, Dentistry and Nursing, University of Glasgow, UK

Introduction

According to World Health Organization global estimates, more than a million of people each day acquire a sexually transmitted infection (STI), with the highest burden being in low-income countries [1]. The burden of STI has major consequences including suffering from the infection itself and adverse health outcomes impacting on the individual's physical and mental health [2]. Health-related consequences of STIs include foetal and neonatal death, cervical and oropharyngeal cancer, infertility, increased risk of another STI [2], low self-esteem [3] and stigma. In addition, there are social and economic consequences. Individuals with STIs often face discrimination, indifference and sometimes hostility even in healthcare settings [4].

STIs were historically diagnosed in public health clinics for reasons of anonymity, confidentiality, contact tracing, and specialised care [5]. In recent years, most reported cases are from service providers in non-STI clinics, such as private physician's offices and community health centres [6].

Prevention is a key component in the control of sexually transmitted diseases [5]. Strategies to prevent STIs include male latex condoms, behavioural counselling, pre-exposure vaccination and presumptive treatment after exposure [7,8]. Center for Disease Control and Prevention (CDC)'s *Sexually Transmitted Diseases Treatment Guidelines (2015)* provide clinical guidance to healthcare providers on the prevention, diagnosis and treatment of STIs [7].

Barriers to Effective Prevention and Care of STIs

Factors that hinder the effective prevention and treatment of STIs are discussed by the United Nations Program on HIV/AIDS (UNAIDS) under the following categories.

- *Many STIs are asymptomatic*: Asymptomatic individuals especially women do not know that they have an STI and hence will not seek care. They will continue to be infected and infectious to others [9].
- *Reluctance to seek healthcare:* Even with symptoms, some infected people may be reluctant to seek care. This can be out of ignorance, embarrassment or guilt. They may also be deterred by an unfriendly attitude of healthcare staff, a lack of privacy or confidentiality, or an intimidating setting [9].
- *Failure to notify spouse or sex partner(s):* Patients may not inform their sex partners about the infection out of fear, embarrassment or unawareness of the importance of doing so [9].
- *Unavailability or unsuitability of sexual health services:* sexual health services may not exist in a particular locality. Even where they exist, they may be difficult to access, especially for women and young people, or they may lack privacy or confidentiality. Patients may be deterred from attending by the stigma attached to dedicated sexual health clinics. Rectal infection may not be recognised in men who have sex with men [9].
- *Patient ignorance of STIs:* Ignorance or misinformation about the causes, symptoms, cures and consequences of STIs and human immunodeficiency virus (HIV)/acquired immune deficiency syndrome (AIDS) is widespread, particularly among adolescents and young people. This population is likely to be sexually active, unlikely to be in stable sexual relationships, and have poor access to sexual health services [9].
- *Substandard treatment:* Although treatment for syphilis, gonorrhoea, chlamydial infection, chancroid, and trichomoniasis is effective when the correct drugs are given, cheaper but substandard treatments may be prescribed in an effort to save money. This practice perpetuates infection and may lead to the emergence of resistant organisms [9].

STI Prevention and Care

The objectives of sexual health services are to reduce the prevalence of STIs, reduce the duration of infection and prevent their complications [7–9].

- Primary prevention aims to protect healthy individuals from acquiring an infection by promoting safe sex (including barrier methods), performing vaccination, and providing information and education [8]
- Secondary prevention aims to eliminate symptoms and prevent complications. The main tools of secondary prevention of STIs are early diagnosis, prompt treatment, and contact tracing to identify and treat sexual partners [8].

- Treatment cures many infections and interrupts the chain of transmission by rendering the patient non-infectious even with incurable viral infections such as HIV [8].

The Clinician's Role

Healthcare providers in various disciplines can play a key role by taking a sexual history, assessing risk for STIs, performing screening and diagnostic testing, providing on-site medications, and notifying and managing sex partners [5,7,10].

Sexual History

The healthcare provider should consider the individual's risk factors for disease acquisition, the possibility of transmission and the likelihood of progression to clinically significant disease [11–14]. Variables include age, sexuality (heterosexual, homosexual or bisexual), sexual behaviours, the clinical circumstances, gender power dynamics within the relationship, local disease prevalence, cultural norms and healthcare-seeking behaviour [12]. Healthcare providers are encouraged to obtain sexual histories from their patients at initial and follow-up visits whether or not it seems relevant to the chief complaint [11]. They should ask about the number of sex partners, gender of sex partners and specific sexual practices (oral, vaginal or anal sex) [5]. Women who have sex with women (WSW) are at risk of acquiring STIs from current or prior male and female partners [12]. Counselling and screening recommendations for WSW are the same as those applicable for men having sex with men (MSM) [12].

Physical examination of a patient with STI-related symptoms includes inspection of the skin, mouth, pharynx, lymph nodes, anogenital area and nervous system [9].

Screening and diagnostic testing are used to detect an asymptomatic infection or confirm a suspected infection [5].

Notifying and treating sex partners interrupts transmission, prevents re-infection of the index case, and might prevent complications from unrecognised infection in the partner [5].

The CDC has defined '5 Ps' as an interactive counselling technique (Box 4.1) [11].

Box 4.1   Interactive '5 P s' Counselling Method

The 5Ps

1) **P**artners: Men, women or both? Lifetime partners? Current partners? Monogamy?
2) **P**revention of pregnancy: What are you doing to prevent pregnancy?
3) **P**rotection from STIs: How do you protect yourself against STIs?
4) **P**ractices: Vaginal, anal oral sex? Condoms?
5) **P**ast History of STIs (in patient or patient's partners)

Source: Adapted from Centers for Disease Control and Prevention [11].

Clinic-Based Interventions for STI Prevention

Healthcare providers should explain how STIs can be prevented. Some approaches include the following.

Abstinence

The most effective way of preventing an STI is the avoidance of oral, vaginal and anal sex, as contact between body parts and fluids facilitates pathogenic transmission [9,12].
   When abstinence is not feasible, the following methods are recommended.

- *Condoms:* Condoms are physical barriers to infection and impermeable to STI pathogens. Providers should counsel patients about consistent and correct use of condoms for penetrative sex acts to maximise their effectiveness. A new condom should be used throughout every act of oral, vaginal and anal sex [5,7,9–11]. Dental dams are effective in preventing transmission of STIs during oral–vaginal and oral–anal sex [12].
- *Reduction in the number of sex partners:* Delay in sexual initiation and a reduction in the number of lifetime partners may reduce an individual's risk of acquiring an STI. Both partners are recommended to undergo STI screening prior to the initiation of any sexual contact and prior to resuming contact if one of the partners has had sexual relations with another individual [12].
- *Immunisation:* Pre-exposure vaccination for human papillomavirus (HPV), hepatitis A and hepatitis B is highly effective at preventing transmission of these viruses. In many countries, girls and boys are offered HPV vaccination ideally before the first sexual contact. However, there is considerable variation in guidelines internationally. Both hepatitis A and hepatitis B vaccines are recommended by the CDC for all men who have sex with men and for anyone using illicit intravenous drugs [7]. A combined hepatitis A and hepatitis B vaccine (Twinrix) is now available [9,11,12].
- *Pre-exposure prophylaxis:* HIV pre-exposure prophylaxis (PrEP) is highly effective in reducing HIV acquisition among gay and bisexual men who adhere to the medication plan [13]. PrEP does not protect against other STIs.

Patients should be told that many STIs are not detectable immediately after exposure and that some STIs, particularly latent viruses like herpes simplex virus (HSV) may be difficult to detect [12]. It is critical that individuals undergoing treatment for an STI should be abstinent until the completion of medical therapy to reduce the chance of transmitting the infection and being reinfected [9,12].

Partner Management

When a patient is diagnosed with an STI, the healthcare provider should promote treatment of infected partners to stop further disease's transmission [9,12]. Patients diagnosed with an STI should be told to disclose this to their partners and urge them to seek testing and treatment.

Referral to a Specialist

Patients with a complex STI or STI-related condition should be referred to a clinician who has specialised training or experience in diagnosing and treating STIs [5].

Role of Oral Healthcare Providers in STI Prevention

STIs and the Mouth

Anyone exposed to an infected partner can get an STI in the mouth, throat, genitals or rectum [15]. Throughout the world, oral sex among young adults has increased in recent years [16]. The risk of acquiring an STI or transmitting an STI to others through oral sex depends on the particular STI, the type of sex and the number of sex acts performed. Using a condom, dental dam or another barrier method at every oral sex act can reduce the risk. Receptive oral sex from a partner with a mouth or throat infection may transmit an STI to the anogenital region [15]. Oral sex involving the anus can transmit hepatitis A and B [15]. Oral healthcare providers can play a key role in prevention and educating the public about the risks involved with oral sex.

- *Discussing sexual history with dental patients:* A sexual history should be taken when there are oral symptoms and signs suggestive of STIs. Dental patients may not be at ease talking about their sexual history, sex partners or sexual practices with their oral health professionals. However, the CDC guidelines [14] for physicians can easily be adapted for the dental practice for patients who present with an oral lesion suspected to be syphilis (chancre), HPV infection (condyloma acuminatum and oropharyngeal carcinoma), or HIV disease (Kaposi sarcoma or an oral opportunistic infection in an otherwise healthy adult).

Oral healthcare providers could use the following dialogue:

> "Sexually transmitted infections can be related to oral health. When examining mouth of every adult patient, I look for signs of sexually transmitted infections. In this regard, I would like to ask you a few questions about your sexual health and sexual practices. I understand that these questions are very personal, but they are important for your overall health as well as your oral health. I routinely ask these questions to adult patients, regardless of age, gender or marital status. This information is kept in strict confidence. Do you have any questions before we get started?"

Examination, Referral and Patient Education

Oral healthcare providers should monitor for lesions suspicious of STIs and provide proper counsel and referral if they suspect infection.

Dental practitioners should be aware of the oral manifestations of gonorrhoea, syphilis, viral warts, infectious mononucleosis, genital herpes, chlamydia and trichomoniasis, which have a high incidence among the general population. Delayed treatment of these diseases can lead to sterility and pelvic inflammatory disease. Ulcers increase the risk of HIV infection [7,9,11,12,17–20] (see Chapters 10–17.) Refer to the local specialty clinic where available. Dental practitioners may also need to instruct patients on safe sexual behaviour, medical treatment of infected partners and the risks of sharing needles [20].

A Special Note on HPV Infection

The popularity of oral sex among young adults has led to an increase in HPV 16 infection and HPV-associated oropharyngeal cancers [16]. Oral healthcare providers should talk to patients and their parents about the prevention of oral HPV infection and oropharyngeal cancer by HPV vaccination.

Dental practitioners should consider having brochures about the HPV vaccination available in their treatment and reception rooms, and give educational materials to at-risk patients and their parents. CDC recommends that females through the age of 26 and males through the age of 21 should be vaccinated [17]. However, as previously mentioned, there is significant variation internationally.

According to a study from the American Association for Cancer Research, poor oral health, including gum disease, was found to be an independent risk factor for oral HPV infection [18]. Men and women aged 30–69 years old, who reported poor oral health, had a 56% higher prevalence of oral HPV infection than those with good oral health. The study concluded, 'Given that oral hygiene is fundamental for oral health and that it is modifiable, public health interventions may aim to promote oral hygiene and oral health as additional preventive measures for HPV-related oral cancers [19]'.

Infection Control in Dental Setting

Creation of safe healthcare environments through the implementation of evidence-based infection control practices that minimise the risk of transmission of infectious agents is an essential requirement for all dental settings. Standard precautions are the basic processes of infection prevention and control. Dental staff should be aware of the national guidelines on infection control. When a contaminated sharps injury occurs to a staff member, it is followed up correctly with baseline tests of that injured staff member [21].

References

1 World Health Organization (2013). *The Importance of a Renewed Commitment to STI Prevention and Control in Achieving Global Sexual and Reproductive Health.* Geneva: WHO.

2 Joint United Nations Programme on HIV/AIDS, World Health Organization (2013). *Sexually Transmitted Diseases: Policies and Principles for Prevention and Care.* Geneva: World Health Organization http://www.who.int/hiv/pub/sti/en/prev_care_en.pdf.

3 Gardner, L.H., Frank, D., and Amankwaa, L.I. (1998). A comparison of sexual behavior and self-esteem in young adult females with positive and negative tests for sexually transmitted diseases. *ABNF J.* 9 (4): 89–94. pmid:9987212.

4 Garcia, P.J., Miranda, A.E., Gupta, S. et al. (2021). The role of sexually transmitted infections (STI) prevention and control programs in reducing gender, sexual and STI-related stigma. *EClin. Med.*, ISSN: 2589-5370 33: 100764.

5 Barrow, R.Y., Ahmed, F., Bolan, G.A., and Workowski, K.A. (2020). Recommendations for providing quality sexually transmitted diseases clinical services, 2020. *MMWR Recommen. Rep.* 68 (5): 1–20. https://doi.org/10.15585/mmwr.rr6805a1.

6 Center for Disease Control and Prevention (CDC) (2019). *Sexually Transmitted Disease Surveillance 2018*. Atlanta: US Department of Health and Human Services https://www .cdc.gov/std/stats18/default.htm.

7 Workowski, K.A. and Bolan, G.A. (2015). Centers for Disease Control and Prevention. Sexually transmitted diseases treatment guidelines, 2015. *MMWR Recommend. Rep.* 64 (RR-031): 1–137.

8 Suligoi, B., Giuliani, M., and Le, M.S.T. (2000). STDs today: risk groups and prevention tools. *Minerva Ginecol.* 52 (12 Suppl 1): 1–6.

9 The public health approach to STD control: UNAIDS Technical Update (1998). (UNAIDS Best Practice Collection: Technical Update). Geneva.

10 Wimberly, Y.H., Hogben, M., Moore-Ruffin, J. et al. (2006). Sexual history-taking among primary care physicians. *J. Natl. Med. Assoc.* 98: 1924–1929.

11 Centers for Disease Control and Prevention (2010, 2010). Sexually transmitted diseases treatment guidelines. *MMWR* 59 (RR-12): 1–110.

12 Moniz, M.H. and Beigi, R.H. (2012). Prevention of sexually transmitted diseases. In: *Sexually Transmitted Diseases*. Chapter 17 (ed. R.H. Beigi), 161–170. UK: Wiley.

13 Traeger, M.W., Cornelisse, V.J., Asselin, J. et al. (2019). Association of HIV preexposure prophylaxis with incidence of sexually transmitted infections among individuals at high risk of HIV infection. *JAMA* 321 (14): 1380–1390. https://doi.org/10.1001/jama.2019.2947.

14 Centre for Disease Control and Prevention (CDC) (2020). A Guide to Taking a Sexual History: https://www.cdc.gov/std/treatment/sexualhistory.pdf

15 Centre for Disease Control and Prevention CDC (2021). STD Risk and Oral Sex | STD|CDC. https://www.cdc.gov/std/healthcomm/stdfact-stdriskandoralsex.htm

16 Nguyen, N.P., Nguyen, L.M., Thomas, S. et al. (2016, 2016). Oral sex and oropharyngeal cancer. *Medicine* 95 (28): e4228. https://doi.org/10.1097/MD.0000000000004228.

17 Centers for Disease Control and Prevention (2018). HPV vaccine information for clinicians. HPV vaccine recommendations. https://www.cdc.gov/hpv/hcp/need-to-know.pdf.

18 American Dental Association (2019). Oral health and HPV infection. American Association for Cancer Research Journal. https://www.colgate.com/en-us/oral-health/ conditions/hiv-aids-and-STIs/ada-08-study-examines-oral-health-hpvi-infection. Published 2019. Accessed January 16, 2019

19 Bui, T.C., Markham, C.M., Ross, M.W., and Mullen, P.D. (2013). Examining the association between oral health and oral HPV infection. *Cancer Prev. Res.* 6 (9): 917–924. http://dx.doi .org/10.1158/1940-6207.CAPR-13-0081. http://cancerpreventionresearch.aacrjournals.org/ content/6/9/917.

20 Angus, J., Langan, S.M., Stanway, A. et al. (2006). The many faces of secondary syphilis: a re-emergence of an old disease. *Clin. Exp. Dermatol.* 31: 741–745.

21 Australian Dental Association (2021). *Guidelines for Infection Prevention and Control*, 4e. Australia: St Leonards NSW.

5

Human Immunodeficiency Virus Infection and Acquired Immunodeficiency Syndrome (HIV/AIDS): An Overview

S.R. Prabhu[1] and Nicholas van Wagoner[2]

[1]University of Queensland, School of Dentistry, Brisbane, Australia
[2]Department of Infectious Diseases, University of Alabama at Birmingham, Heersink School of Medicine, Birmingham, Alabama, USA

Glossary of HIV/AIDS Related Terms

A glossary of human immunodeficiency virus (HIV)-related terms is provided to define the words that are commonly used to describe the virus that causes HIV disease, its pathogenesis, clinical manifestations, diagnosis, treatment and prevention.

Acquired Immunodeficiency Syndrome (AIDS): AIDS is the most advanced stage of HIV infection. To be diagnosed with AIDS, a person with HIV must have an AIDS-defining condition or have a CD4 count less than 200 cells mm^{-3} (regardless of whether the person has an AIDS-defining condition).

Antiretroviral Therapy (ART): It is the combination of HIV medicines (called an HIV regimen) used to treat HIV infection. A person's initial HIV regimen generally includes three antiretroviral (ARV) drugs from at least two different HIV drug classes.

Chemokine Receptor 5 (CCR5): This is a protein on the surface of certain immune system cells, including CD4 T lymphocytes (CD4 cells). CCR5 can act as a co-receptor (a second receptor binding site) for HIV when the virus enters a host cell.

Cell-Mediated Immunity: Type of immune response that is produced by the direct action of immune cells, such as T lymphocytes, rather than by antibodies.

Chemokines: Small proteins secreted by cells to mobilise and activate infection fighting white blood cells. Chemokines are involved in many immune and inflammatory responses.

Cytokines: A family of proteins produced by cells, especially by immune cells. Cytokines act as chemical messengers between cells to regulate immune responses.

Deoxyribonucleic Acid (DNA): One of two types of genetic material found in all living cells and many viruses. DNA carries the genetic instructions for the development and function of an organism. DNA allows for the transmission of genetic information from one generation to the next.

Sexually Transmissible Oral Diseases, First Edition.
Edited by S.R. Prabhu, Nicholas van Wagoner, Jeff Hill and Shailendra Sawleshwarkar.
© 2023 John Wiley & Sons Ltd. Published 2023 by John Wiley & Sons Ltd.

Entry Inhibitor: A group of antiretroviral HIV drugs that include fusion inhibitors, CCR5 antagonists, and post-attachment inhibitors. Entry inhibitors block HIV from entering a host CD4 cell.

Epidemic: A widespread outbreak of a disease affecting a large number of individuals over a particular period of time either in a given area or among a specific group of people.

False Negative: A test result that incorrectly indicates that the condition being tested for is not present when, in fact, the condition is actually present. For example, a false-negative HIV test indicates that a person does not have HIV, but the person actually does have HIV.

False Positive: A test result that incorrectly indicates that the condition being tested for is present when, in fact, the condition is actually not present. For example, a false-positive HIV test indicates that a person has HIV, but the person actually does not have HIV.

Fusion Inhibitor: A fusion inhibitor blocks the HIV envelope from merging with the host CD4 cell membrane (fusion). This prevents HIV from entering the CD4 cell.

Gene Therapy: Manipulating genes to treat or prevent disease. Gene therapy techniques being researched include replacing a defective gene with a healthy copy of the gene, repairing an abnormal gene, inactivating an improperly functioning gene and introducing a new disease-fighting gene.

Genome: The complete genetic material of an organism, including all of its genes. The genome is contained in a set of chromosomes in humans and in a DNA or RNA molecule in viruses. The HIV genome consists of an RNA molecule and includes nine genes.

gp120: A glycoprotein on the HIV envelope. gp120 binds to a CD4 receptor on a host cell, such as a CD4 cell. This starts the process by which HIV fuses its viral envelope with the host cell membrane and enters the host cell.

gp41: A glycoprotein on the HIV envelope. HIV enters a host cell by using gp41 to fuse the HIV envelope with the host cell membrane.

Humoral Immunity: Type of immune response that is mediated by antibodies.

Hypersensitivity Syndrome: A life-threatening allergic reaction to a drug. Hypersensitivity syndrome is characterised by fever, rash, organ involvement (most frequently, the liver) and high blood levels of oeosinophils. Use of certain ARV drugs may cause hypersensitivity syndrome.

Immunodeficiency: Inability to produce an adequate immune response because of an insufficiency or absence of antibodies, immune cells or both. Immunodeficiency disorders can be inherited, such as severe combined immunodeficiency; they can be acquired through infection, such as with HIV, or they can result from chemotherapy and immunosuppressive therapy used for the treatment of autoimmune disorders and other diseases and used after organ transplant to prevent organ rejection.

Immunosuppression: When the body's ability to mount an immune response to fight infections or disease is reduced. Immunosuppression may be caused by certain diseases, such as HIV, or by radiotherapy or chemotherapy. Immunosuppression may also be deliberately induced by drugs used to prevent rejection of transplanted organs.

Immunotherapy: Use of immunologic agents such as antibodies, growth factors and vaccines to modify (activate, enhance or suppress) the immune system in order to treat disease. Immunotherapy is also used to diminish adverse effects caused by some cancer treatments or to prevent rejection of a transplanted organ or tissue.

Incidence: The number of new cases of a condition, symptom, death or injury that develops in a specific area during a specific period of time.

Integrase: An enzyme found in HIV (and other retroviruses). HIV uses integrase to insert (integrate) its viral DNA into the DNA of the host CD4 cell. Integration is a crucial step in the HIV life cycle and is blocked by a class of antiretroviral HIV drugs called integrase strand transfer inhibitors (INSTIs).

Lentivirus: A subgroup of retroviruses, which includes HIV.

LGBTQ: Acronym for lesbian, gay, bisexual, transgender and questioning/queer.

Messenger RNA (mRNA): A type of RNA that carries the genetic information needed to make a protein

MSM: Acronym for men who have sex with men

MSMW: Acronym for men who have sex with men and women

Mutation: A permanent change in the genetic material of a cell or microorganism. Some mutations can be transmitted when the cell or microorganism replicates. Some HIV mutations cause the virus to become resistant to certain ARV drugs.

Occupational Post-Exposure Prophylaxis (oPEP): Short-term treatment started immediately after high-risk occupational exposure to an infectious agent, such as HIV, hepatitis B virus (HBV) or hepatitis C virus (HCV). An example of a high-risk occupational exposure is exposure to an infectious agent as the result of a needle–stick injury in a healthcare setting. The purpose of occupational oPEP is to reduce the risk of infection.

Opportunistic Infection (OI): An infection that occurs more frequently or is more severe in people with weakened immune systems, such as people with HIV or people receiving chemotherapy or other immunosuppressants, than people with healthy immune systems.

p24: A major protein contained in HIV's viral core.

Pneumocystis Jirovecii Pneumonia: Formerly known as Pneumocystis carinii pneumonia. A lung infection caused by the fungus *Pneumocystis jirovecii.*

Polymerase Chain Reaction (PCR): A laboratory technique used to produce large amounts of a specific DNA fragment from a sample that contains very tiny amounts of that DNA. PCR is used for genetic testing and to diagnose disease.

Post-Exposure Prophylaxis (PEP): Short-term treatment started immediately after high-risk exposure to an infectious agent, such as HIV, HBV or HCV. The purpose of PEP is to reduce the risk of infection.

Pre-Exposure Prophylaxis (PrEP): An HIV prevention method for people who are HIV negative and at high risk of HIV infection. PrEP involves taking a specific combination of HIV medicines daily. PrEP is even more effective when it is combined with condoms and other prevention tools.

Protease: A type of enzyme that breaks down proteins into smaller proteins or smaller protein units, such as peptides or amino acids. HIV protease cuts up large precursor proteins into smaller proteins. These smaller proteins combine with HIV's genetic material to form a new HIV virus. Protease inhibitors (PIs) prevent HIV from replicating by blocking protease.

Protease Inhibitor (PI): Antiretroviral HIV drug class. PIs block protease (an HIV enzyme). By blocking protease, PIs prevent new (immature) HIV from becoming a mature virus that can infect other CD4 cells.

Provirus: An inactive viral form that has been integrated into the genes of a host cell. For example, when HIV enters a host CD4 cell, HIV RNA is first changed to HIV DNA (provirus). The HIV provirus then gets inserted into the DNA of the CD4 cell. When the CD4 cell replicates, the HIV provirus is passed from one cell generation to the next, ensuring ongoing replication of HIV.

Rapid Test: A type of HIV test used to screen for HIV infection. A rapid HIV antibody test can detect HIV antibodies in blood or oral fluid in less than 30 minutes. There is also a rapid antigen/antibody test available. A positive rapid HIV test must be confirmed by a second test for a person to be definitively diagnosed with HIV infection [1].

Recombinant: DNA produced in a laboratory by joining segments of DNA from different sources. Recombinant can also describe proteins, cells or organisms made by genetic engineering.

Retrovirus: A type of virus that uses RNA as its genetic material. After infecting a cell, a retrovirus uses an enzyme called reverse transcriptase to convert its RNA into DNA. The retrovirus then integrates its viral DNA into the DNA of the host cell, which allows the retrovirus to replicate. HIV is a retrovirus.

Reverse Transcriptase (RT): An enzyme found in HIV (and other retroviruses). HIV uses RT to convert its RNA into viral DNA, a process called reverse transcription. Non-nucleoside reverse transcriptase inhibitors (NNRTIs) prevent HIV from replicating by blocking RT.

Reverse Transcription: A step in the HIV replication cycle. Once inside a CD4 cell, HIV releases and uses reverse transcriptase (an HIV enzyme) to convert its genetic material – HIV RNA – into HIV DNA. The conversion of HIV RNA to HIV DNA allows HIV to enter the CD4 cell nucleus and combine with the cell's genetic material – cell DNA.

Ribonucleic Acid (RNA): One of two types of genetic material found in all living cells and many viruses. There are several types of RNA. RNA plays important roles in protein synthesis and other cell activities.

Seroconversion: The transition from infection with HIV to the detectable presence of HIV antibodies in the blood. When seroconversion occurs (usually within a few weeks of infection), the result of an HIV antibody test changes from HIV negative to HIV positive.

Sensitivity: The probability that a medical test will detect the condition being tested in people who actually have the condition. In other words, a sensitive test is one that produces true positive results. For example, the enzyme-linked immunosorbent assay (ELISA) HIV antibody test is highly sensitive, which means the test can detect HIV in most people. However, because the ELISA test can sometimes mistakenly recognise antibodies to other diseases as antibodies to HIV (a false-positive result), another HIV test is used to confirm a positive ELISA HIV antibody test.

Specificity: The probability that a medical test will correctly produce a negative test result for a person who does not have the condition being tested. In other words, a specific test is the one that produces true negative results.

Viral Load (VL): The amount of HIV in a sample of blood. VL is reported as the number of HIV RNA copies per millilitre of blood. An important goal of antiretroviral therapy is to suppress a person's VL to an undetectable level – a level too low for the virus to be detected by a VL test.

Window Period: The time period from exposure to HIV infection to when the body produces enough HIV antigen or antibodies to be detected by standard HIV tests. The length of the window period varies depending on the test used. During the window period, a person can have a negative result on an HIV test despite having HIV.

(Modified from: AIDS info Glossary of HIV AIDS-related terms (2018) 9th Edition. The US Department of Health and Human Services (HHS))

Introduction

In the four decades since the human immunodeficiency virus (HIV) and acquired immunodeficiency syndrome (AIDS) were first identified, there has been a phenomenal amount of research on their aetiopathogenesis, transmission, clinical course, diagnosis, treatment and prevention. A large number of reports on oral lesions in HIV disease have also been published in the literature. Evidence confirms that oral lesions in people living with HIV/AIDS can often be early manifestations of HIV-associated immune deficiency. Often these lesions serve as first signs of the underlying HIV infection. Oral lesions in these patients can also become clinical markers of disease progression and often provide information on the adverse effect of antiretroviral drugs, treatment failure, or non-adherence of therapy. Basic knowledge of HIV and AIDS enables oral healthcare practitioners to suspect the presence of disease in their patients early and provides patients with opportunities for receiving appropriate referral, therapy, support and education on preventing its transmission. This chapter is intended to provide an overview of HIV/AIDS. Detailed description of oral lesions in HIV/AIDS is provided in Chapter 11.

Epidemiology

Origin and Global Statistics

AIDS was first recognised as a new disease in 1981 when an increased number of young gay men succumbed to unusual opportunistic infections and rare malignancies [2, 3].

In 1981, a few cases of Kaposi's sarcoma and pneumocystis carinii pneumonia (now known as pneumocystis jirovecii pneumonia) were reported among gay men in New York and California. It was not until mid-1982 that scientists realised that the 'disease' was also spreading among other populations such as people with haemophilia and who inject heroin. By September that year, the 'disease' was named acquired immunodeficiency syndrome (AIDS) [4, 5]. In 1983, the virus now known as HIV was isolated and identified [6–8]. This virus was initially referred to as human T-lymphotropic virus type III (HTLV-III) or lymphadenopathy-associated virus (LAV) [5]. It is widely believed that HIV is the result of an animal-to-human (zoonotic) transfer of a simian immunodeficiency virus (SIV) from primates in Africa [8].

According to UNAIDS Global HIV and AIDS statistics (2022), 84.2 million of people have become infected with HIV since the start of the epidemic and 40.1 million people have died from AIDS-related illnesses [9, 10]. Globally, about 38.4 million of people were living with HIV in 2021 and 1.5 million people became newly infected with HIV [9]. Sub-Saharan Africa acounts for more than two-thirds of all people living with HIV globally. In this region, a greater proportion of women than men is living with HIV and women continue to suffer high rates of new infection. In this region, females aged 15–24 years are twice as likely to be living with HIV and six in seven new HIV infections among adolescents aged 15–19 years are in females. Both social (including health inequities) and biological factors contribute to the vulnerability to HIV among women in Sub-Saharan Africa [11]. Parts of Asia and the Pacific follow next in number of persons living with HIV. The Caribbean as well as Eastern Europe are also heavily affected [10].

While AIDS related deaths have declined substantially over the last 20 years, they still remain high. In 2021, around 650,000 deaths worldwide were attributed to HIV (www. unaids.org/en/resources/fact-sheet). In addition, HIV has indirectly contributed to morbidity and mortality from other infections. It has led to a resurgence of tuberculosis (TB), particularly in Africa, and TB is a leading cause of death for people with HIV worldwide. In 2019, approximately 9% of new TB cases occurred in people living with HIV. However, between 2000 and 2019, TB deaths in people living with HIV declined substantially, largely due to the scale up of joint HIV/TB services. UNAIDS 2021 global data also show that people living with HIV experience more severe outcomes and have higher comorbidities from COVID-19 than those living without HIV [12]. In mid-2021, most people living with HIV did not have access to COVID-19 vaccines. Studies from England and South Africa have found that the risk of dying from COVID-19 among people with HIV was double that of the general population [13, 14].

Key Populations

Key populations are defined groups who, due to specific behaviours, are at increased risk of HIV irrespective of the epidemic type or local context. Legal and social inequities related to their behaviours contribute to their increased vulnerability to HIV [15]. Key populations include sex workers and their clients, gay, bisexual, and other men who have sex with men (MSM), people who inject drugs (PWID), transgender people and their sexual partners. They account for 70% of HIV infections globally, 94% of new HIV infections outside of sub-Saharan Africa, and 51% of new HIV infections in sub-Saharan Africa [9, 15]. Risk for HIV infection is 28 times higher in MSM than men who have sex with women; 35 times higher among PWID than adult who do not inject drugs; 30 times higher for female sex workers than adult women, and 14 time higher for transgender women than cis-gender women (https://www.unaids.org/en/resources/fact-sheet). While key populations have higher rates of HIV, anyone can get HIV [9].

Transmission

Sexual Transmission

The most frequent mode of transmission of HIV is through sexual contact with an infected person. However, an HIV-positive person who has an undetectable viral load as a result of long-term treatment has effectively no risk of transmitting HIV sexually [16].

Likelihood of sexual transmission of HIV depends on several factors including the sex act, the amount of HIV present in the transmitting partner, the presence of STI, the use of barrier protection during sex, and the baseline prevalence of HIV in a person's sexual network. While penile-vaginal sex accounts for most sexual transmissions worldwide, its per-act probability of acquisition through penile-vaginal sex is low compared to penile anal sex. Receptive penile-vaginal intercourse carries a risk of 8 per 10,000 exposures and insertive penile-vaginal intercourse has a probability of acquisition of 4 per 10,000 exposures. In comparison, receptive anal intercourse carries a probability of 138 per 10,000 exposures and a probability of 11 per 10,000 exposures through insertive anal intercourse [17–19]. While transmission is biologically possible through insertive and receptive oral sex, the risk is low, and it is not possible to determine risk per act. Over time, however, repeated even low risk sex increases the likelihood of acquisition [19].

Factors beyond type of sex influence likelihood of HIV acquisition. For example, estimates of the risk of HIV transmission per sexual act appear to be 4–10 times higher in low-income countries than in high-income countries [20]. In low-income countries, the risk of female-to-male transmission is estimated as 0.38% per act and of male-to-female transmission as 0.30% per act; the equivalent estimates for high-income countries are 0.04% per act for female-to-male transmission and 0.08% per act for male-to-female transmission [20]. These differences are believed to be the outcome of complex interacting biologic factors, social factors, and underlying HIV prevalence in the community [21–25]. For example, in setting involving sex work in low-income countries, the risk of female-to-male transmission has been estimated as 2.4% per act and that of male-to-female transmission as 0.05% per act [20]. Risk of transmission also increased in the presence of many sexually transmitted infections (STIs) [26] and genital ulcers [20]. Genital ulcers appear to increase the risk approximately fivefold [20]. Other STIs, such as gonorrhoea, chlamydia, trichomoniasis and bacterial vaginosis, are associated with somewhat smaller increases in risk of transmission [25].

The viral load of an infected person is an important risk factor in sexual transmission [27]. During the first 2.5 months of HIV infection, a person's infectiousness is 12 times higher than that of a person who has had time to mount some immune response to HIV due to the unopposed high viral load associated with acute HIV [25]. As the immune system is damaged by HIV and a person enters the late stage of infection, infectiousness increases and rates of transmission are approximately eight fold of those earlier in infection [20, 28, 29]. Sexual practices that lead to trauma to the genitals, rectum, or mouth can be a factor associated with an increased risk of HIV transmission [30]. Sexual assault is also believed to carry an increased risk of HIV transmission as condoms are rarely worn; physical trauma to the vagina or rectum is likely; and there may be a greater risk of concurrent STIs [30].

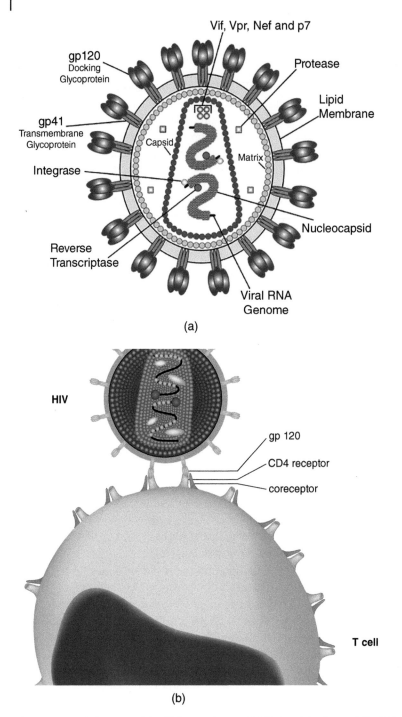

Figure 5.1 (a) Diagram of the HIV virus. (Image: US National Institute of Health). (b) Attachment of gp120 to CD4 cell receptor and chemokine co-receptor.

Other Routes of Transmission

The virus can also be transmitted during the birth process or during breastfeeding [31], via sharing contaminated needles, syringes and other injecting equipment and drug solutions when injecting drugs, when receiving unscreened blood transfusions or tissue transplantation [32], during procedures that involve unsterile cutting, or piercing and through accidental needle stick injuries. Transmission by needle–stick injury occurs in 0.3% of exposures from individuals with HIV infection [33]. Transmission by blood products is now exceedingly rare in countries where blood is screened.

Virology/Pathogenesis

HIV belongs to the genus *Lentivirus*, which is a part of the Retroviridae family. Two types of HIV have been characterised: HIV-1 and HIV-2. HIV-1 is the virus that was originally discovered (and initially referred to as LAV or HTLV-III) [6, 8, 34]. It is more virulent and more infective, and is the cause of the majority of HIV infections globally. HIV-1 can be further subdivided into different groups (M, O and N) and genetic subtypes.

HIV is a single-stranded ribonucleic acid (RNA) virus with an outer envelope that surrounds two copies of single-stranded RNA and a number of viral proteins [8, 34] (Figure 5.1). From its outer envelope protrudes glycoprotein 120 (gp 120). HIV also encodes *Vif, Vpr, Vpu and Nef* as accessory proteins (genes). These accessory proteins help in the efficiency of viral replication. The HIV replication cycle commences when gp 120 attaches to the CD4 receptor (Figure 5.1b) and chemokine co-receptor (chemokine receptor 5, CCR5) [34, 35]. These receptors are expressed on the surface of the CD4 lymphocyte, the cell that HIV predominantly infects. Attachment precipitates the fusion of the viral envelope with the cell membrane via the HIV envelope glycoprotein 41 (gp 41), allowing the virus to enter the cell [34, 35]. The viral RNA then undergoes reverse transcription, a process by which RNA is converted into deoxyribonucleic acid (DNA) using the viral-encoded reverse transcriptase. The resulting viral DNA, called the provirus, migrates to the nucleus and integrates into the host chromosome. The provirus acts as a template to allow the messenger RNA to produce the components of new virus particles, including the RNA genome of new virions [34–36]. The viral proteins are processed and cleaved by another virus-specific enzyme known as HIV protease. Viral proteins and RNA are then assembled and bud from the cell membrane, forming mature HIV particles that can infect other cells [35–38]. Some of the CD4 cells are irreparably damaged by HIV infection. Premature cell death of damaged CD4 cells in part contributes to the immunosuppression characteristic of advanced HIV disease.

Typical Course of Untreated HIV Infection

Acute HIV infection, also known as early or primary HIV infection, is a condition that develops within two to four weeks of contracting HIV. The time after infection and before seroconversion, during which markers of infection (p24 antigen and antibodies) are still absent or too scarce to be detectable, is called the window period. Screening tests cannot always detect HIV infection during the window period [35, 39–41].

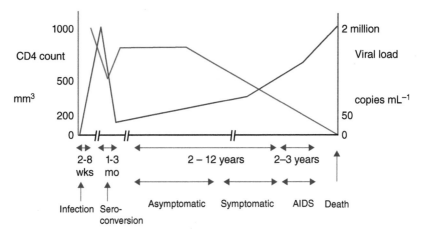

Figure 5.2 Typical course of untreated HIV infection. Source: HIV i-Base (2016) How CD4 and Viral Load are Related. Treatment training manual. https://i-base.info/ttfa/section-2/14-how-cd4-and-viral-load-are-related.

Within 12–24 hours, HIV infects cells at the site of exposure (i.e., genital, anal, or oral mucosa). By forty-eight hours after exposure, HIV has spread to regional lymph nodes where rapid replication occurs within immune cells, primarily CD4 cells. Cells in the gut become infected as well as those of the central nervous system and the skin [35, 39–41]. Over the next 5–40 days, the host immune response to massive HIV viraemia results in the production of antibodies, and a cytotoxic T-cell response mounted by CD8$^+$ T lymphocytes [35, 39–41]. The T-helper CD4 cells not only control the cytotoxic response but also are infected by HIV. Early in the course of infection, memory CD4$^+$ cells are selectively depleted from the circulation. As disease advances, both naive cells (CD4 cells with very little capacity to mount an immune response) and memory phenotype CD4 cells are lost [35, 39–41]. Factors such as cellular destruction, diminished cellular production and cellular sequestration in lymphoid tissue cause the characteristic depletion of lymphocytes in HIV disease. The number of circulating CD4$^+$ lymphocytes is used as a measure of immune competence. This provides a predictor of risk for opportunistic illnesses. The changes in immune function as a result of HIV infection can be observed by monitoring CD4 and CD8 cell counts in the peripheral blood [35, 39–41]. The flu-like symptoms of acute HIV infection are thought to be caused by the release of cytokines during the process of infection and immune response. As a result of the immune response, the blood concentration of the virus (the viral load) falls, and new CD4 cells are produced by the bone marrow via the thymus. The cytotoxic CD8 cells and antibody responses are not able to clear or completely control HIV replication [35, 39–41]. Figure 5.2 shows typical course of untreated HIV infection.

Clinical Features

Signs and Symptoms of Acute HIV Infection

Signs and symptoms of acute HIV infection (primary infection) can present as early as 3 days or as late as 10 weeks following infection. Most commonly, they occur at 10–14 days

The onset of symptoms often coincides with the appearance of HIV antibodies, although the patient may be HIV antibody negative for up to three weeks after the onset of symptoms. The duration of this illness is most commonly 4–14 days but may be longer. Approximately 50–90% of patients report signs or symptoms suggestive of acute HIV infection at the time of seroconversion. During this time, antibody tests may be negative for HIV, but the serum viral load is detectable and can be quite high (millions of copies per millilitre) [42–45]. The frequency of symptoms varies and severity ranges from mild to severe. Although no single symptom distinguishes acute HIV infection from other acute viral illnesses, there are some factors that should alert the clinician to the possibility of acute HIV infection. These include 'glandular fever-like' illness, 'flu-like' symptoms including myalgia, arthralgia, headache, malaise, illness of sudden onset, pharyngitis and fever for more than three days [42–45]. Persistent generalised lymphadenopathy (PGL) is often the earliest symptom of acute HIV infection. Because of marked follicular hyperplasia in response to HIV infection, the lymph nodes have very high viral concentrations. Oral thrush from *Candida* infection, oral hairy leukoplakia due to Epstein–Barr virus (EBV) infection and aphthous stomatitis can occur during this stage of the disease (for oral manifestations, see Chapter 11). Other features include maculopapular rash, meningeal involvement and transient neurological syndromes or genital ulcers. Thrombocytopenia may be an early manifestation of HIV infection. 10–20% of patients infected with HIV may manifest reactivation of varicella-zoster virus (shingles). Oral and genital herpes simplex lesions are also common [42–45]. Patients presenting with any symptoms consistent with acute HIV should undergo a complete sexual and social history to characterize the likelihood of HIV as the cause.

Chronic HIV Infection and AIDS

This begins after antibodies to the virus are fully developed and the initial immune response is complete [43–45]. Although the symptoms of acute HIV resolve, continued viral replication leads to progressive damage to the immune system. The rate of damage to the immune system and progression toward AIDS directly correlates with HIV RNA levels. Individuals with high levels of HIV RNA progress to AIDS faster than patients with low levels of HIV RNA. Some individuals develop symptoms or organ dysfunction during chronic infection due to direct effects of the virus rather than to immune system damage. Some infected persons, who are otherwise asymptomatic, develop PGL during this time [43–45].

AIDS is the condition that results from long-term (chronic) HIV infection and is defined by an absolute CD4 cell count of less than 200 cells μL^{-1} and/or the presence of specific opportunistic infections or malignancies [43–45]. The interval between acute HIV infection and AIDS is highly variable. In the absence of specific treatment, around 50% of people infected with HIV develop AIDS within 10 years. The most common initial conditions that alert to the presence of AIDS are pneumocystis pneumonia, cachexia in the form of HIV wasting syndrome and oesophageal candidiasis. Other common signs include recurrent respiratory tract infections. People with AIDS have an increased risk of developing various viral-induced cancers, including Kaposi's sarcoma, Burkitt's lymphoma, primary central nervous system lymphoma and cervical cancer [43–45].

HIV and TB

HIV has led to a resurgence of TB, particularly in Africa, and TB is a leading cause of death for people with HIV worldwide. However, between 2000 and 2019, TB deaths in people living with HIV declined substantially, largely due to the scale up of joint HIV/TB services [46].

Diagnosis

The history should be carefully taken to elicit possible exposures to HIV. While no physical findings are specific to HIV, HIV infection should be considered in patients with unusual or recurrent serious infections without another cause, especially in those who have risk factors for HIV infection. Generalised lymphadenopathy and weight loss are common. Evidence for risk factors or minor concurrent opportunistic infections such as herpetic lesions on the groin or widespread oral candidiasis (see Chapter 9) may provide clues to HIV infection. Most people infected with HIV develop specific antibodies within 3–12 weeks after the initial infection.

Diagnosis of primary HIV before seroconversion is done by measuring HIV-RNA or p24 antigen. HIV/AIDS is diagnosed via laboratory testing and then staged based on the presence of certain signs and symptoms [47–49]. The length of time between exposure and reliable detection of infection, called window period, depends on the virus population dynamics and the types of laboratory tests applied.

Investigations

When history and/or clinical presentation indicate the possibility of acute, chronic, or advanced HIV (i.e., AIDS) infection, laboratory testing ensures correct diagnosis. HIV infection is identified either by the detection of HIV-specific antibodies in serum or plasma or by demonstrating the presence of the virus by nucleic acid detection using polymerase chain reaction (PCR) or p24 antigen testing. Antibodies to HIV can be measured by a variety of techniques [47–49]. Antibody testing is the method most commonly used to diagnose HIV infection. Antibody tests do not detect HIV itself, but rather detect the immune response to the virus, and therefore take some time to develop and become reactive (or positive) after HIV infection. Antibodies to HIV-1 and HIV-2 are detected by enzyme-linked immunosorbent assay (ELISA), simple/rapid test devices and western blot (WB) tests [47–49]. HIV antibody tests (HIV ELISA and western blot) may be negative up to three weeks after the start of symptoms associated with acute HIV. Re-testing is strongly recommended in patients with an HIV risk event in the 12 weeks preceding a negative antibody test result. In the context of acute HIV infection, the use of rapid HIV antibody tests is not appropriate for diagnostic purposes, as these tests are insensitive when antibody titres are low. However, HIV viraemia appears in the blood about 10 days after infection and allows for direct detection of virus particles or proteins (antigens) in the absence of antibodies. Tests for viral antigens facilitate earlier diagnosis of HIV infection. Tests that detect viral RNA or antigen should therefore be considered confirmatory (of an indeterminate serology result) when used in this setting [47–49]. Combined antigen/antibody tests (also known as fourth generation tests) are also available and used by many laboratories for HIV screening.

Rapid HIV Testing

Traditional HIV testing, where blood is drawn and sent to the laboratory for testing, can take several days or more to get a result. Rapid testing uses a pinprick of the finger (or oral fluid, depending on the test) and returns results within 10–20 minutes. Most rapid HIV tests detect HIV antibodies; however, some can also test for the presence of the virus itself [49, 50]. A 'reactive' (or preliminary positive) result on a rapid HIV test does not diagnose HIV, as rapid HIV tests produce a small number of false-positive results [49, 50]. For this reason, a reactive rapid HIV test result must always be confirmed by laboratory tests. HIV self-testing (also known as home-based testing) kits are also available where HIV testing is conducted in the home or similar environment.

Treatment

There is currently no cure for HIV. The aim of therapy for HIV infection is to sustain an undetectable viral load and to produce immune reconstitution [51–53]. According to the Guidelines for the use of antiretroviral agents in Adults and Adolescents with HIV, Antiretroviral therapy (ART) is recommended for all persons with HIV to reduce morbidity and mortality and to prevent the transmission of HIV to others [54]. Similarly, the World Health Organization recommends ART initiation in all adults with HIV regardless of WHO clinical stage and at any CD4 cell count. While this is the goal, feasibility of this recommendation may differ by country. Therefore, the WHO recommends prioritizing ART in adults with severe or advanced HIV clinical disease (WHO clinical stage 3 or 4) and adults with CD4 counts less than or equal to 350 cells/mm^3.

Highly Active Antiretroviral Therapy and Combination Antiretroviral Therapy

The course of HIV has been drastically altered by the introduction of highly active antiretroviral therapy (HAART) or combination antiretroviral therapy (cART). This therapy usually consists of a combination of at least three drugs from two or three of the different classes of antiretroviral drugs [52, 53]. Classes of drugs used include the nucleoside analogue reverse transcriptase inhibitors (NRTIs), the non-nucleoside reverse transcriptase inhibitors (NNRTIs), protease inhibitors (PIs), integrase inhibitors (II), fusion inhibitors, gp 120 attachment inhibitors and CCR5 antagonists. A combination of three agents, usually two NRTIs combined with either an NNRTI or PI or II, are used to suppress HIV viral replication and treat HIV. Antiretroviral drug classes are discussed below [52, 53].

NRTIs

NRTIs force the HIV virus to use faulty versions of building blocks so that infected cells cannot produce more HIV. This class of drugs include abacavir or ABC (Ziagen), didanosine or ddI (Videx), emtricitabine or FTC (Emtriva), lamivudine or 3TC (Epivir), stavudine or d4T (Zerit), tenofovir alafenamide or TAF (Vemlidy), Tenofovir disoproxil fumarate or TDF (Viread) and zidovudine or ZDV (Retrovir) [51–53].

NNRTIs

NNRTIs bind to a specific protein, so that the HIV virus becomes unable to make copies of itself. This group of drugs include delavirdine or DLV (Rescripor), doravirine or DOR (Pifeltro), efavirenz or EFV (Sustiva), etravirine or ETR (Intelence), nevirapine or NVP (Viramune) and rilpivirine or RPV (Edurant) [51–53].

Protease Inhibitors

Protease inhibitors work by interfering with HIV enzymes that cleave precursor proteins and are necessary for production of infectious viral particles. This group includes atazanavir or ATV (Reyataz), darunavir or DRV (Prezista), fosamprenavir or FPV (Lexiva), indinavir or IDV (Crixivan), lopinavir + ritonavir or LPV/r (Kaletra), nelfinavir or NFV (Viracept), ritonavir or RTV (Norvir), saquinavir or SQV (Invirase and Fortovase) and tipranavir or TPV (Aptivus) [51–53].

Integrase Inhibitors

Integrase inhibitors stop HIV from making copies of itself by blocking a key protein, which allows the virus to put its DNA into the DNA of a healthy cell. These are also called integrase strand transfer inhibitors (INSTIs). Drugs in this class include bictegravir or BIC, cabotegravir (Vocabria), dolutegravir or DTG (Tivicay), elvitegravir or EVG (Vitekta) and raltegravir or RAL (Isentress) [51–53].

Fusion Inhibitors

Unlike NRTIs, NNRTIs, PIs, and INSTIs, which work on infected cells, fusion inhibitors block HIV from getting inside healthy cells. These include enfuvirtide or ENF or T-20 (Fuzeon) [51–53].

gp120 Attachment Inhibitor

This is a new class of drug with just one medication, fostemsavir (Rukobia). This is for adult patients who have tried multiple HIV medications and whose HIV is resistant to other therapies. It targets gp 120 on the surface of the virus, stopping it from being able to attach itself to the CD4 T cells of the body's immune system [51–53].

CCR5 Antagonist

Maraviroc or MVC (Selzentry) stops HIV before it gets inside a healthy cell, but in a different way than fusion inhibitors. It blocks a specific kind of 'hook' on the outside of certain cells so the virus cannot plug in [52, 53].

Combination ART

Combination HIV pills (cART) are available that contain 2 or more antiretroviral medications from one or more drug classes. These combination pills greatly improve adherence resulting in improved HIV outcomes. More than 20 combination pills are manufactured worldwide and the number continues to grow [55].

Side Effects of Antiretroviral Drugs

Many of the antiretroviral drugs have significant side effects, and some have complex dosing schedules, making adherence an issue for concern [56, 57]. However, fixed-dose combination drugs are now available, and most of the newer antiretroviral agents are administered once or twice daily, making adherence to combination regimens easier. Long-term survival has also unmasked chronic drug toxicities, particularly metabolic problems such as lipodystrophy and lipoatrophy, hyperlipidaemia, insulin resistance and hepatic mitochondrial toxicity [57]. However, with new medications, side effects and drug toxicities are infrequent and ART is well-tolerated.

Prognosis

HIV/AIDS has become a chronic manageable infection rather than a fatal disease. Prognosis varies between people, and both the CD4 count and viral load are useful for predicting outcomes. Without treatment, average survival time after infection with HIV is estimated to be 9–11 years, depending on the HIV subtype. After the diagnosis of AIDS, if treatment is not available, survival ranges between 6 and 19 months [57, 58]. Many variables have been implicated in HIV's rate of progression, CCR5-delta32 heterozygosity, mental health, concomitant drug or alcohol abuse, superinfection with another HIV strain, nutrition and age [57, 58]. The primary causes of death from HIV/AIDS are opportunistic infections and cancer both of which are frequently the result of the progressive failure of the immune system. TB co-infection is one of the leading causes of sickness and death in those with HIV/AIDS present in a third of all HIV-infected people and causing 25% of HIV-related deaths [57, 58].

Prevention

Individuals can reduce the risk of HIV infection by limiting exposure to risk factors. Key approaches for HIV prevention, which are often used in combination, include use of condoms by both men and women, testing and counselling for HIV and STIs, testing and counselling for linkages to TB care, voluntary medical male circumcision (VMMC), use of antiretroviral drugs (ARVs) for prevention, harm reduction for people who inject and use drugs, and elimination of mother-to-child transmission of HIV [59–61].

Recent Risk of Exposure

Patients reporting recent risk of exposure should be thoroughly assessed and monitored for HIV infection. Patients reporting an occupational HIV exposure (nurses, doctors, dentists, dental nurses, chiropodists, ambulance officers, police officers and others) or a non-occupational HIV risk event (such as unprotected anal or vaginal intercourse; shared injecting equipment or other exposure to potentially infectious body fluids where the source is known or likely to have HIV infection) and the exposure has occurred within the previous 72 hours should be considered for HIV post-exposure prophylaxis (PEP) [59–61].

Post-Exposure Prophylaxis

Post-exposure prophylaxis (PEP) is a preventive strategy that aims to prevent an actual or potential exposure to HIV from becoming an infection following non-occupational exposure, e.g. condom less sexual contact, shared injecting equipment in PWID (non-occupational PEP or NPEP) or in healthcare workers occupationally exposed to HIV (occupational PEP or OPEP) [59, 60, 62–64].

PEP comprises a 28-day course of three antiretroviral drugs commenced within 72 hours of exposure. PEP efficacy is time dependent; therefore, it is essential that assessment and referral be made as early as possible within the 72-hour period since exposure. Effective implementation also requires thorough medical assessment of the exposed individual and source (where possible); an informed estimation of the HIV transmission risk related to the exposure; baseline testing for blood-borne viruses; clinical and laboratory follow-up; and the provision of information, risk reduction counselling and support. Potential exposure to HIV often indicates a risk of HBV and HCV infection as well as a risk of other STIs. Consequently, investigations for STIs prevalent in the community, HBV and HCV should be considered in any person being assessed for HIV post-exposure prophylaxis [62–64].

The 2016 PHS guidelines for antiretroviral post-exposure prophylaxis for non-occupational exposure to HIV recommend either RAL 400 mg twice daily or DTG 50 mg daily in combination with TDF 300 mg and FTC 200 mg daily as the preferred regimen in healthy adults and adolescents [64].

Pre-Exposure Prophylaxis for Non-HIV-Infected People

Pre-exposure prophylaxis (PrEP) should be considered for the non-HIV-infected individuals. These individuals include [65–68]:

- Anyone who is in an ongoing sexual relationship with an HIV-infected partner.
- A gay, bisexual, or other man who has sex with men without a condom or has been diagnosed with a sexually transmitted infection within the past six months and is not in a mutually monogamous relationship with a partner who recently tested HIV negative.
- A heterosexual man or woman who does not always use condoms when having sex with partners known to be at risk for HIV and who is not in a mutually monogamous relationship with a partner who recently tested HIV negative.
- Anyone who, in the preceding six months, has injected illicit drugs and shared equipment or been in a treatment program for injection drug use.

Prevention of Mother-to-Child Transmission

Programmes to prevent the vertical transmission of HIV (from mothers to children) can reduce rates of transmission by 92–99%. This primarily involves the use of a combination of antiviral medications during pregnancy and after birth in the infant, and potentially includes bottle feeding rather than breast feeding [69].

Patient Education

Patients with HIV infection should be counselled about the risks of infecting their sexual partners with HIV. Safer sex practices and treatment of concurrent sexually transmitted infections, both in the patient and in sexual partners, considerably reduce the risk of transmission. Patients with HIV infection should be encouraged to inform their sexual partners about their status; In some countries it is required by law to share HIV status. Patients should be made aware of such laws as needed [70].

Vaccine Against HIV

The initial hope of an effective vaccine against HIV has not been fulfilled. The greatest challenge in developing an effective HIV vaccine has been the high rate of mutation and recombination during viral replication. Aside from the virus being able to rapidly mutate antigenic portions of key surface proteins, HIV infection progresses despite the host's humoral and cellular immune responses; therefore, any vaccination effect needs to surpass the normal host response to HIV [71–73].

References

1 Recommended Laboratory HIV Testing Algorithm for Serum or Plasma Specimens (2014). https://www.cdc.gov/hiv/pdf/guidelines_testing_recommendedlabtestingalgorithm.pdf.

2 CDC (1981). Kaposi's sarcoma and pneumocystis pneumonia among homosexual men – New York City and California. *MMWR Morb. Mortal. Wkly. Rep.* 30: 305–308.

3 Greene, W.C. (2007). A history of AIDS: looking back to see ahead. *Eur. J. Immunol.* 37 (Suppl. 1): S94–S102.

4 Brennan, R.O. and Durack, D.T. (1981). Gay compromise syndrome. *Lancet* 2 (8259): 1338–1339.

5 Reeves, J.D. and Doms, R.W. (2002). Human immunodeficiency virus type 2. *J. General Virol.* 83 (6): 1253–1265. https://doi.org/10.1099/0022-1317-83-6-1253. PMID 12029140.

6 Broder, S. and Gallo, R.C. (1984). A pathogenic retrovirus (HTLV-III) linked to AIDS. *N. Engl. J. Med.* 311 (20): 1292–1297. https://doi.org/10.1056/NEJM198411153112006. PMID: 6208484.

7 Barré-Sinoussi, F., Chermann, J.C., Rey, F. et al. (1983). Isolation of a T-lymphotropic retrovirus from a patient at risk for acquired immune deficiency syndrome (AIDS). *Science.* 220 (4599): 868-71. doi: 10.1126/science.6189183. PMID: 6189183.

8 Sharp, P.M. and Hahn, B.H. (2010). The evolution of HIV-1 and the origin of AIDS. *Philos. Trans. R. Soc. B Biol. Sci.* 365 (1552): 2487–2494. https://doi.org/10.1098/rstb.2010.0031. ISSN 09628436. PMC 2935100. PMID 20643738.

9 Global HIV & AIDS statistics — Fact sheet 2022. https://www.unaids.org/sites/default/files/media_asset/UNAIDS_FactSheet_en.pdf.

10 Govender, R.D., Hashim, M.J., Khan, M.A. et al. (2021). Global epidemiology of HIV/AIDS: a resurgence in North America and Europe. *J. Epidemiol. Hlobal Health* 11 (3): 296–301. https://doi.org/10.2991/jegh.k.210621.001.

11 Sia, D., Onadja, Y., Hajizadeh, M. et al. What explains gender inequalities in HIV/AIDS prevalence in sub-Saharan Africa? Evidence from the demographic and health surveys. BMC Public Health 16, 1136 (2016). https://doi.org/10.1186/s12889-016-3783-5.

12 UNAIDS 2021. https://www.unaids.org/en/resources/presscentre/featurestories/2021/october/20211011_people-living-with-hiv-covid19.

13 Geretti, A.M., Stockdale, A.J., Kelly, S.H. et al. (2021). Outcomes of Coronavirus Disease 2019 (COVID-19) Related Hospitalization Among People With Human Immunodeficiency Virus (HIV) in the ISARIC World Health Organization (WHO) Clinical Characterization Protocol (UK): A Prospective Observational Study. *Clin. Infect. Dis.* 73(7): e2095-e2106. doi: 10.1093/cid/ciaa1605. PMID: 33095853; PMCID: PMC7665382.

14 Western Cape Department of Health in collaboration with the National Institute for Communicable Diseases, South Africa (2021). Risk Factors for Coronavirus Disease 2019 (COVID-19) Death in a Population Cohort Study from the Western Cape Province, South Africa. *Clin. Infect. Dis.* 73(7): e2005-e2015. doi: 10.1093/cid/ciaa1198. Erratum in: Risk Factors for Coronavirus Disease 2019 (COVID-19) Death in a Population Cohort Study from the Western Cape Province, South Africa. (2022). *Clin. Infect. Dis.* 74(7): 1321. PMID: 32860699; PMCID: PMC7499501.

15 Consolidated Guidelines on HIV Prevention, Diagnosis, Treatment and Care for Key Populations – 2016 Update. Geneva: World Health Organization; 2016. DEFINITIONS OF KEY TERMS. Available from: https://www.ncbi.nlm.nih.gov/books/NBK379697/.

16 LeMessurier, J., Traversy, G., Varsaneux, O. et al. (2018). Risk of sexual transmission of human immunodeficiency virus with antiretroviral therapy, suppressed viral load and condom use: a systematic review. *Can. Med. Assoc. J.* 190 (46): E1350–E1360. https://doi.org/10.1503/cmaj.180311. PMC 6239917. PMID 30455270.

17 HIV Risk Behaviors. https://www.cdc.gov/hiv/risk/estimates/riskbehaviors.html

18 Centers for Disease Control and Prevention (CDC) (2019). HIV and Men. U.S. Department of Health & Human Services. https://www.cdc.gov/hiv/group/gender/men/index.html

19 Centers for Disease Control and Prevention (2019). HIV and All Gay and Bisexual Men. U.S. Department of Health & Human Services. https://www.cdc.gov/hiv/group/msm/index.html

20 Boily, M.C., Baggaley, R.F., Wang, L. et al. (2009). Heterosexual risk of HIV-1 infection per sexual act: systematic review and meta-analysis of observational studies. *Lancet Infect. Dis.* 9 (2): 118–129. https://doi.org/10.1016/S1473-3099(09)70021-0. PMC 4467783. PMID 19179227.

21 Beyrer, C., Baral, S.D., van Griensven, F. et al. (2012). Global epidemiology of HIV infection in men who have sex with men. *Lancet* 380 (9839): 367–377. https://doi.org/10.1016/S0140-6736(12)60821-6. PMC 3805037. PMID 22819660.

22 Yu, M. and Vajdy, M. (2010). Mucosal HIV transmission and vaccination strategies through oral compared with vaginal and rectal routes. *Expert Opin. Biol. Therapy* 10 (8): 1181–1195. https://doi.org/10.1517/14712598.2010.496776. PMC 2904634. PMID 20624114.

23 Stürchler, D.A. (2006). *Exposure a Guide to Sources of Infections*, 544. Washington, DC: ASM Press.

24 Pattman, R., Sankar, N., Elawad, B. et al. (ed.) (2010). *Oxford Handbook of Genitourinary Medicine, HIV, and Sexual Health*, 2e, 95. Oxford: Oxford University Press.

25 Dosekun, O. and Fox, J. (2010). An overview of the relative risks of different sexual behaviours on HIV transmission. *Curr. Opin. HIV AIDS* 5 (4): 291–297. https://doi.org/10.1097/COH.0b013e32833a88a3. PMID 20543603. S2CID 25541753.

26 Ng, B.E., Butler, L.M., Horvath, T., and Rutherford, G.W. (2011). Population-based biomedical sexually transmitted infection control interventions for reducing HIV infection. *Cochrane Database System. Rev.* (3): CD001220. https://doi.org/10.1002/14651858.CD001220.pub3. PMID 21412869.

27 Anderson, J. (2012). Women and HIV: motherhood and more. *Curr. Opin. Infect. Dis.* 25 (1): 58–65. https://doi.org/10.1097/QCO.0b013e32834ef514. PMID 22156896. S2CID 6198083.

28 Kerrigan, D. (2012). *The Global HIV Epidemics among Sex Workers*, 1–5. World Bank Publications.

29 Aral, S. (2013). *The New Public Health and STD/HIV Prevention: Personal, Public and Health Systems Approaches*, 120. Springer.

30 Klimas, N., Koneru, A.O., and Fletcher, M.A. (2008). Overview of HIV. *Psychosomatic Med.* 70 (5): 523–530. https://doi.org/10.1097/PSY.0b013e31817ae69f. PMID 18541903. S2CID 38476611.

31 UNAIDS (1998). Mother-to-child transmission of HIV. https://www.unaids.org/sites/default/files/media_asset/jc531-mtct-tu_en_0.pdf

32 Simonds, R.J. (1993). HIV transmission by organ and tissue transplantation. *AIDS* 7 (Suppl 2): S35–S38. https://doi.org/10.1097/00002030-199311002-00008. PMID 8161444. S2CID 28488664.

33 Centers for Disease Control and Prevention (2019). HIV Risk Behaviors | HIV Risk and Prevention Estimates. https://www.cdc.gov/hiv/risk/estimates/riskbehaviors.html

34 HIV, Viral Hepatitis and STIs – A Guide for Primary Health CareDanta, M. and Wray, L. (2014, 2014. Chapter 1). HIV, HBV, HCV and STIs: Similarities and Differences. In: , 7–24. Melbourne: Australasian Society for HIV Medicine (ASHM).

35 German Advisory Committee Blood-Subgroup (2016). 'Assessment of pathogens transmissible by blood' – human immunodeficiency virus (HIV). *Transfusion Med. Hemotherapy* 43 (3): 203–222. https://doi.org/10.1159/000445852.

36 Demirkhanyan, L., Marin, M., Lu, W., and Melikyan, G.B. (2013). Sub-inhibitory concentrations of human α-defensin potentiate neutralizing antibodies against HIV-1 gp41 pre-hairpin intermediates in the presence of serum. *PLoS Pathog.* 2013 (9): e1003431.

37 Maher, D., Wu, X., Schacker, T. et al. (2005). HIV binding, penetration, and primary infection in human cervicovaginal tissue. *Proc. Natl. Acad. Sci. U.S.A.* 102: 11504–11509.

38 Levy, J.A. (2011). Virus-host interactions in HIV pathogenesis: directions for therapy. *Adv. Dent. Res.* 23: 13–18.

39 Jaffar, S., Grant, A.D., Whitworth, J. et al. (2004). The natural history of HIV-1 and HIV-2 infections of adults in Africa: a literature review. *Bull. World Health Organ.* 82: 462–469.

40 HIV i-Base (2016). How CD4 and Viral Load are Related. Treatment training manual. https://i-base.info/ttfa/section-2/14-how-cd4-and-viral-load-are-related

41 Zablotska, I., McAllister, J., Keen, P. et al. (2014). Exposure and acute HIV infection (Chapter 4). In: *HIV, Viral Hepatitis and STIs – A Guide for Primary Care* (ed. M. Burke, T. Cabrie, B. Cowie, et al.), 49–56. Sydney: Australasian Society for HIV Medicine (ASHM).

42 Kelleher, A.D. and Cooper, D.A. (2008). *Acute HIV Infection, Global HIV/AIDS Medicine*, 63–74. Elsevier.

43 Baliga, C.S., Mary, E., Javier, P. et al. (2008). HIV infection and acquired immunodeficiency syndrome. In: *Clinical Immunology (Third Edition). Principles and Practice* (ed. R.R. Rich, T.A. Fleisher, W.T. Shearer, et al.), 561–584. Elsevier.

44 World Health Organization (2007). *WHO Case Definitions of HIV for Surveillance and Revised Clinical Staging and Immunologic Classification of HIV-Related Disease in Adults and Children*, 1–48. Geneva, Switzerland: World Health Organization.

45 HIV i-Base (2019) The natural history of HIV in detail. Guide. https://i-base.info/guides/art-in-pictures/the-natural-history-of-hiv-in-detail

46 Fry, S.H.-L., Barnabas, S.L., and Cotton, M.F. (2019). Tuberculosis and HIV – an update on the "cursed duet" in children. *Front. Pediatr.* https://doi.org/10.3389/fped.2019.00159.

47 Fearon, M. (2005). The laboratory diagnosis of HIV infections. *Can. J. Infect. Dis. Med. Microbiol.* 16 (1): 26–30. https://doi.org/10.1155/2005/515063.

48 Sax, P.E. (2021). Screening and diagnostic testing for HIV infection. UpToDate. https://www.uptodate.com/contents/screening-and-diagnostic-testing-for-hiv-infection

49 Cennimo, D.J. (2021). HIV testing Overview. Medscape reference. https://emedicine.medscape.com/article/2061077-overview

50 Isserman, J.D. (2021). Rapid HIV testing: Overview. Medscape. https://emedicine.medscape.com/article/783434-overview

51 Eisinger, R.W., Dieffenbach, C.W., and Fauci, A.S. (2019). HIV viral load and transmissibility of HIV infection: undetectable equals untransmutable. *JAMA* 321 (5): 451–452. https://doi.org/10.1001/jama.2018.21167. PMID 30629090. S2CID 58599661.

52 US Department of Health and Human Services. (2015). Guidelines for the Use of Antiretroviral Agents in HIV-1-Infected Adults and Adolescents.

53 Simon, V., Ho, D.D., and Abdool Karim, Q. (2006). HIV/AIDS epidemiology, pathogenesis, prevention, and treatment. *Lancet* 368 (9534): 489–504. https://doi.org/10.1016/S0140-6736(06)69157-5. PMC 2913538. PMID 16890836.

54 Guideline on When to Start Antiretroviral Therapy and on Pre-Exposure Prophylaxis for HIV. Geneva: World Health Organization; 2015 Sep. PMID: 26598776. https://clinicalinfo.hiv.gov/en/guidelines/hiv-clinical-guidelines-adult-and-adolescent-arv/initiation-antiretroviral-therapy?view=full

55 FDA-Approved HIV Medicines. https://hivinfo.nih.gov/understanding-hiv/fact-sheets/fda-approved-hiv-medicines

56 Info HIV (2021). Adverse effects of antiretroviral drugs. https://clinicalinfo.hiv.gov/en/guidelines/adult-and-adolescent-arv/adverse-effects-antiretroviral-agents

57 Gilroy, S.A. (2020). What is the prognosis of untreated HIV infection? https://www.medicinenet.com/hiv_treatment_drugs_prognosis_and_prevention/views.htm

58 Poorolajal, J., Hooshmand, E., Mahjub, H. et al. (2016). Survival rate of AIDS disease and mortality in HIV-infected patients: a meta-analysis. *Public Health* 139: 3–12. https://doi.org/10.1016/j.puhe.2016.05.004. Epub 2016 Jun 24. PMID: 27349729.

59 HIV info (2021). The Basics of HIV Prevention. https://hivinfo.nih.gov/understanding-hiv/fact-sheets/basics-hiv-prevention

60 Spach, D.H. and Kalapila, A.G. (2021). Preventing HIV Transmission in Persons with HIV. National HIV curriculum Modules. University of Washington (2nd edition). https://www.hiv.uw.edu/go/prevention

61 Zablotska, I., McAllister, J., and McNulty, A. (2014). Biomedical prevention of HIV. In: *HIV, Viral Hepatitis and STIs – A Guide for Primary Health Care*, 169–179. Melbourne: Australasian Society for HIV Medicine (ASHM).

62 Ana Elizabeth Markelz (2021). Postexposure HIV Prophylaxis in Physicians and Medical Personnel. Medscape. https://emedicine.medscape.com/article/1991375-overview.

63 ASHM (2016). National Guidelines for Post-Exposure Prophylaxis after non-Occupational and Occupational Exposure to HIV (second Edition). pp. 4–22. www.ashm.org.au/resources/PEP_GUIDELINES_2016.FINAL_ONLINE_VERSION.pdf

64 Kuhar, D.T. et al. (2018). Updated U.S. Public Health Service guidelines for the management of occupational exposures to HIV and recommendations for postexposure prophylaxis. USPHS Working Group on Occupational Postexposure Prophylaxis.; National Center for Emerging and Zoonotic Infectious Diseases (U.S.). Division of Healthcare Quality Promotion. Published Date: 9/25/2013 Update (May 23, 2018). https://stacks.cdc.gov/view/cdc/20711

65 Grulich, A.E., Guy, R., Amin, J. et al. (2018). Population-level effectiveness of rapid, targeted, high-coverage roll-out of HIV pre-exposure prophylaxis in men who have sex with men: the EPIC-NSW prospective cohort study. *Lancet HIV* 2018 (5): e629–e637.

66 Mayer, K.H., Molina, J.M., Thompson, M.A. et al. (2020). Emtricitabine and tenofovir alafenamide vs emtricitabine and tenofovir disoproxil fumarate for HIV pre-exposure prophylaxis (DISCOVER): primary results from a randomised, double-blind, multicentre, active-controlled, phase 3, non-inferiority trial. *Lancet* 396 (10246): 239–254. https://doi.org/10.1016/S0140-6736(20)31065-5.

67 Bhatti, O., So, D., Zahid, M.A., and Cornelisse, V.J. (2021). Prescribing pre-exposure prophylaxis in general practice. *Aust. J. General Pract.* 50: 479–482.

68 Grant, R.M., Anderson, P.L., McMahan, V. et al. (2014). Uptake of pre-exposure prophylaxis, sexual practices, and HIV incidence in men and transgender women who have sex with men: a cohort study. *Lancet Infect. Dis.* 14 (9): 820–829. https://doi.org/10.1016/S1473-3099(14)70847-3.

69 Dong, Y., Guo, W., Gui, X. et al. (2020). Preventing mother to child transmission of HIV: lessons learned from China. *BMC Infect. Dis.* 20: 792. https://doi.org/10.1186/s12879-020-05516-3.

70 UNAIDES (2014). Charting the course of education and HIV. https://www.unaids.org/en/resources/presscentre/featurestories/2014/april/20140401unesco

71. Gray, G.E., Laher, F., Lazarus, E. et al. (2016). Approaches to preventative and therapeutic HIV vaccines. *Curr. Opin. Virol.* 17: 104–109. https://doi.org/10.1016/j.coviro.2016.02.010. PMC 5020417. PMID 26985884.

72. Ditse, Z., Mkhize, N.N., Yin, M. et al. (2020). Effect of HIV envelope vaccination on the subsequent antibody response to HIV infection. *mSphere* 5: 1–13. https://doi.org/10.1128/mSphere.00738-19.

73. Nguni, T., Chasara, C., and Ndhlovu, Z.M. (2020). Major Scientific Hurdles in HIV Vaccine Development: Historical Perspective and Future Directions. Frontiers in Immunology. {https://www.frontiersin.org/article/10.3389/fimmu.2020.590780}

Section 2

The Mouth and the Risky Sexual Behaviours

6

Defence Mechanisms of Oral and Genital Mucosae

Pallavi Hegde[1], Raghavendra Rao[1], S.R. Prabhu[2], and Sujitha Reddy[1]

[1]*Department of Dermatology, Kasturba Medical College, Manipal, India*
[2]*University of Queensland, School of Dentistry, Brisbane, Australia*

Introduction

The skin and orogenital mucosae are the body's first line of defence and offer protective barriers against infection. Being the point of entry to the gastrointestinal and genitourinary tract, respectively, oral and genital mucosae are at risk of developing various sexually transmitted infections (STIs). Oral and genital mucosal contact is common in fellatio and cunnilingus. This type of sexual activity often results in transmitting STIs from an infected partner to a non-infected partner. It is not uncommon to encounter sexually acquired infections in oral and genital mucosae simultaneously. Under normal circumstances, oral and genital mucosae resist the pathogenic microbial invasion by virtue of their protective mechanisms. To understand the pathogenesis of sexually transmitted diseases, clinicians should possess basic knowledge of the mucosal defence mechanisms involved against microbial invasion.

Oral Mucosa

Mucous membrane is the lining of the oral cavity. It extends from vermillion border of the lips to the anterior pillars of the fauces. Histologically, it consists of an outermost surface epithelium that is of a stratified squamous type and an underlying zone of fibrous connective tissue [1]. These two compartments are separated by a basement membrane (basal lamina). The deeper layer of the epithelium projects deep into lamina propria as undulating projections, known as rete pegs, and interdigitate with papillary projections of the lamina propria. The oral mucosa is contiguous with deeper connective tissues – the submucosa [1, 2]. This structure contains neurovascular tissues, lymphatics, adipose tissue and minor salivary gland tissue at certain sites [1–3]. The mucosal epithelium is a

Sexually Transmissible Oral Diseases, First Edition.
Edited by S.R. Prabhu, Nicholas van Wagoner, Jeff Hill and Shailendra Sawleshwarkar.

continuously self-renewing tissue with the rate of renewal of cells varying from site to site in the mouth [4]. Average turn over time for buccal mucosa is 14 days, whereas the same for floor of the mouth and hard palate are 20 and 24 days, respectively [1, 3–5]. Detailed structure and functions of the oral mucosa are beyond the scope of this chapter.

Oral Mucosal Defence Mechanisms

The commensal (resident) microbial populations of the mouth do not cause disease and may keep pathogenic species in check by not allowing them to adhere to mucosal surfaces (see Chapter 7.), In addition, a few other mechanisms operate to protect the oral cavity from the attack of pathogenic microorganisms. These protective mechanisms can be discussed under two headings: non-specific and specific protective mechanisms.

Non-Specific Protective Mechanisms

Non-specific protective mechanisms can broadly be grouped under four categories: surface integrity, bacterial balance, saliva and enzymes, and phagocytic cells and compliment systems [6].

Surface Integrity
The intact surface epithelium supported by lamina propria presents a mechanical barrier to oral microorganisms. The continuous shedding by exfoliation of epithelial squames also limits oral microbial colonisation [3, 6–8]. Mucosal defences are further supported by the membrane coating granules discharged extracellularly in the granular cell layer, transudation of antibodies through the mucosa and the barrier presented by the basement membrane [7, 8]. Epithelial Langerhans cells (LCs, antigen-presenting cells) can process antigens in their major histocompatibility complex (MHC)-class II intracellular compartments. They migrate to the regional lymph nodes to present antigenic peptides to prime naïve helper T cells [3, 9]. The efficiency of the surface barrier is further enhanced by epithelial keratinisation and parakeratinisation. Keratinocytes can produce a variety of cytokines such as IL-1, IL-6 and IL-8. Mucosal cytokines may have pro-inflammatory as well as anti-inflammatory functions to maintain the local homeostasis. An imbalance in the cytokine levels can result in many diseases. Two important cytokines involved in mucosal health are IL1 and IL33. IL-1 facilitates the immune response and inflammation by inducing the expression of many proteins, like chemokines, nitric oxide synthetase and matrix metalloproteinases (MMPs). IL 33 augments T helper cell 2 (Th 2) cytokine-mediated inflammatory immune response upon exposure to micro-organism. Cytokines can also be secreted by macrophages, fibroblasts, dendritic cells (DCs) and mast cells in the oral mucosa [7–9]. Certain cell surface receptors of keratinocytes can recognise pathogen-associated molecular patterns (PAMPs), a part of microbial structure and lead pro-inflammatory cytokine release. These cytokines can induce inflammation to destroy the evading organism [6, 9]. Oral epithelial cells constitutively express the

growth-arrest-specific 6 (GAS6) protein acting via the tyrosin–protein kinase receptor. It upregulates the expression of adhesion molecules in blood vessels and thereby causes extravasation of immune cells, and increases the expression of chemokines and migration of DCs to the lymph nodes. In addition, it also promotes the expression of the pro-inflammatory molecules [6, 9, 10].

The keratinised areas are least permeable, and non-keratinised lining areas such as the floor of the mouth are most permeable. This variation appears to reflect differences in the types of lipid making up the intercellular permeability barrier in the superficial layers of the epithelium. Mucosal permeability helps in easier diffusion of immune cells to pass across the mucosa and provide local immunity. This property also provides better absorption of drugs bypassing the first pass metabolism [2, 6, 9, 10].

Bacterial Balance
The mouth as a whole and various zones in the mouth can be viewed as ecosystems in which a balance exists between the different species of microorganisms and between the microflora and tissues. Some mechanisms involved include microbial interference for microbial binding to epithelial cells, competition for nutrients and release of by-products that are toxic to other microbes [6, 9].

Saliva and Enzymes
Saliva has a mechanical effect of flushing microorganisms from the mucosal surface. Saliva also has important antimicrobial agents. These include immune components such as secretory immunoglobulin A (IgA), and non-specific components such as lactoferrin, lactoperoxidase, lysozyme agglutinins and myeloperoxidase system [6, 8].

Phagocytic and Mucosa-Associated Lymphoid Tissue Systems
Certain cells in the blood stream and in the tissues are capable of engulfing and digesting foreign material. The two most important phagocytic cells are polymorphonuclear leukocytes and macrophages. The polymorphonuclear leukocytes protect the body against acute invasion and have the ability for amoeboid movement and can pass through capillaries and through tissues, including the epithelium. The direction of their movement is determined by tissue damage products, which are chemotactic. Macrophages are cells that start as monocytes and, in the tissue, they become efficient phagocytes, which can digest large foreign particles. The macrophages also take up antigens in the circulating fluid for the presentation of lymphocytes. Phagocytosis is aided by a battery of nine related proteins known as 'complement', which act by immobilising the bacteria or toxins, so that phagocytes can act more effectively in disposing foreign matter [2, 7–10].

The oral immune system is part of an extensive compartmentalised mucosa-associated lymphoid tissue (MALT). MALT refers to small concentrations of lymphoid tissue found across various submucosal membranes of the body. It initiates immune responses to specific antigens encountered [6, 9]. The role of MALT in immunity and the mechanism of destroying (neutralising) the antigen (organism) is shown in Box 6.1.

Box 6.1   Mechanism of Neutralising the Antigen

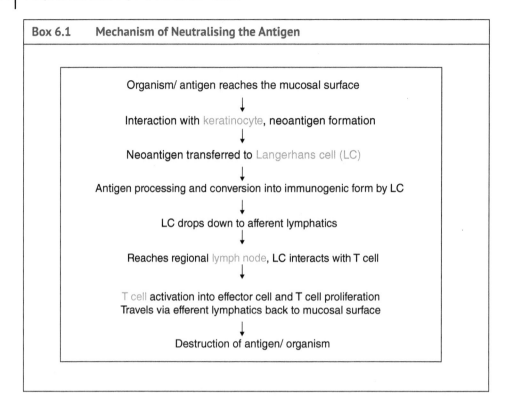

Organism/ antigen reaches the mucosal surface

↓

Interaction with keratinocyte, neoantigen formation

↓

Neoantigen transferred to Langerhans cell (LC)

↓

Antigen processing and conversion into immunogenic form by LC

↓

LC drops down to afferent lymphatics

↓

Reaches regional lymph node, LC interacts with T cell

↓

T cell activation into effector cell and T cell proliferation
Travels via efferent lymphatics back to mucosal surface

↓

Destruction of antigen/ organism

Specific Protective Mechanisms: Humoral and Cellular Immunity

The specific immune system has two basic components: (i) humoral immunity and (ii) cell-mediated immunity, which is separate but inter-dependent. Humoral immunity is mediated through B lymphocyte that has receptors on its surface, which can recognise a specific antigen and promotes B-cell proliferation to become plasma cells, which in turn produce large quantities of special proteins called immunoglobulins, which act as anti-foreign bodies or antibodies. There are five types of immunoglobulins – IgA, IgD, IgE, IgG and IgM. Cell-mediated immunity, on the other hand, is mediated by T lymphocytes, which are circulated constantly in blood and lymph. These take up organisms already active in the body and those which have been taken by macrophages [6, 8, 9].

In summary, mechanisms of oral mucosal defence include (i) physical barriers (epithelium and lamina propria), (ii) non-specific bacterial balance, (iii) saliva containing both non-specific and specific antimicrobial factors and (iv) specific immune humoral and cell-mediated defence mechanisms.

Vaginal Mucosa

The vagina is a fibromuscular structure that connects the cervix to the vulva. It is made up of connective tissue and smooth muscle and is lined by a layer of epithelium.

Histologically, the vaginal mucosa has the following distinct layers from inside to outside [11, 12]:

The first layer is the epithelium, composed of stratified squamous cells with a small amount of keratin, resting on the lamina propria, which is composed of loose connective tissue, a vast number of elastic fibres, giving the vagina its capability to distend, followed by the layer of smooth muscles. The final layer is the adventitia, which is rich in elastic fibres and blood vessels.

The epithelium is folded into involutions called 'rugae' and results in a large surface area of the stratified squamous epithelium, up to $360\,cm^2$ [11]. This increased area puts the women at a higher risk of acquiring STI when exposed to the partner carrying STI infection [12, 13].

Defence Mechanisms of the Vaginal Mucosa

The following factors protect the deeper tissues from pathogenic microorganisms.

- *Physical factors:* Terminally differentiated stratum corneum layer of the vaginal epithelium encases the cells of the epidermis and provides a physical barrier to microorganisms. Cells of the cervix and vaginal epithelium generate a mucous that acts as a barrier and traps the organism [12, 14–16].
- *Immunological factors:* The epithelium is permeable to antibodies and other immune system cells, which in turn prevents the passage of invading pathogens into deeper vaginal tissue. The epithelium also synthesises antimicrobial peptides and immunoglobulins [13, 15].
- *Chemical factors:* The glycogen derived from desquamated cells in the lumen is converted into lactic acid by the bacteria normally resident in the vagina. The resulting acidity is important in protecting the female reproductive tract from infection by pathogenic bacteria [13] (see Chapter 7).
- *Hormonal factors:* Oestrogen stimulates the production of glycogen and maintains the thickness of the epithelium. Before puberty and after menopause when oestrogen levels are relatively low, the epithelium is relatively thin, and the pH is higher than in the reproductive years (neutral prior to puberty and 6.0 or higher after menopause). These factors render females in these groups more susceptible to vaginal infections [13, 16] (see Chapter 7).

Penile Mucosa

The gross structure of the human penis consists of four different regions: (i) the foreskin, a stratified keratinized epithelium, with a highly keratinized outer surface and a less keratinized inner one facing the glans [17], (ii) the glans, covered by stratified keratinized epithelium; (iii) the fossa navicularis (referred to here as fossa), a stratified non-keratinized epithelium, and (iv) the urethra, a pseudo-stratified non-keratinized epithelium [17–19]. Stratified squamous epithelium forms the first later. Epithelium is non-keratinizing at glans penis which becomes keratinized after circumcision. Beneath the epithelium is lamina propria with loose connective tissue and small blood vessels.

Defence Mechanisms of the Penile Mucosa

The susceptibility of penis to STIs depends largely on the intrinsic characteristics of the mucosal immune system of each of different regions of the penile mucosa [19]. The human penis is a main portal of entry for numerous sexually transmitted pathogens such as human papilloma virus (HPV), *Chlamydia trachomatis* or *Neisseria gonorrhoeae*. Human immuno-deficiency virus type 1 (HIV-1) also targets the penile foreskin and urethra.

Mucosal epithelial surfaces are coated with a mucus layer that plays an important role in first-line immune defence by trapping and eliminating microbes before they reach the epithelial surface. Innate and adaptive immune responses also contribute to the protection at mucosal surfaces [19–21]. The mucosal innate immune system offers defence against mucosal pathogens and comprises numerous components including epithelial barriers, anti-microbial peptides [19, 20], pattern recognition receptors, such as toll-like receptors (TLRs) [22], and inflammatory immune cells, such as natural killer (NK) cells and neutro-phils, which are mainly involved in apoptosis of infected cells and phagocytosis, respectively. [20–22]

Antigen-presenting cells that include macrophages, LCs and DCs participate in innate immune responses as well as in the initiation of adaptive immune responses by presenting antigens to lymphocytes. Such adaptive immune responses, which take place in a second step following the innate immune responses, are pathogen specific and involve two arms, namely, the humoral response coordinated predominantly by B cells, with or without CD4$^+$ T cells help, and the cellular response driven by cytotoxic T cells [20–22].

In conclusion, studies on the immunology of the human penile urethra indicate that this mucosal site is immunologically competent and capable of mounting both innate and cellular and humoral adaptive immunological responses [22].

References

1 Wilson, D.F. (2006). Histology of the Oral mucosa. Chapter 27. In: *Textbook of Oral and Maxillofacial Anatomy, Histology And Embryology* (ed. S.R. Prabhu), 157–168. Oxford University Press (Ind).

2 Cruchley, A.T. and Bergmeier, L.A. (2018). Structure and functions of the oral mucosa. In: *Oral Mucosa in Health and Disease* (ed. L. Bergmeier). Cham: Springer https://doi.org/10.1007/978-3-319-56065-6_1.

3 Brizuela, M. and Winters, R. (2021, 2021). Histology, oral mucosa. In: *StatPearls [Internet]*. Treasure Island (FL): StatPearls Publishing.

4 Squier, C. and Brogden, K.A. (2011). The organization of oral mucosa. In: *Human Oral Mucosa: Development, Structure and Function* (ed. C. Squier and K.A. Brogden), 9. 17: Wiley.

5 Squier, C.A. and Kremer, M.J. (2001). Biology of oral mucosa and esophagus. *JNCI Monogr.* 2001: 7–15.

6 Girish, H.C., Sanjay, M., Shyamala, K., and Varsha, V.K. (2016). Oral defense mechanisms. *Res. J. Pharmaceut. Biol. Chem. Sci.* 7: 1947–1962.

7 Cesta, M.F. (2006). Normal structure, function, and histology of mucosa-associated lymphoid tissue. *Toxicol. Pathol.* 34 (5): 599–608.

8 van't Hof, W., Veerman, E.C.I., Nieuw Amerongen, A.V., and Ligtenberg, A.J.M. (2014). Antimicrobial defense systems in saliva. In: *Saliva: Secretion and Functions.* Monograph Oral Science, vol. 24 (ed. L. AJM and V. ECI), 40–51. Basel: Karger.

9 Walker, D.M. (2004). Oral mucosal immunology: an overview. *Ann. Acad. Med. Singapore* 33 (Suppl): 27S–30S.

10 Squier, C. (2011). Functions of oral mucosa. In: *Human Oral Mucosa: Development, Structure and Function* (ed. C. Squier and K.A. Brogden), 1–7. Wiley.

11 Anderson, D.J., Marathe, J., and Pudney, J. (2014). The structure of the human vaginal stratum corneum and its role in immune defense. *Am. J. Reprod. Immunol.* 71 (6): 618–623.

12 Park, Y.J. and Lee, H.K. (2018). The role of skin and orogenital microbiota in protective immunity and chronic immune-mediated inflammatory disease. *Front. Immunol.* https://doi.org/10.3389/fimmu.2017.01955.

13 Boskey, E.R., Cone, R.A., Whaley, K.J., and Moench, T.R. (2001). Origins of vaginal acidity: high d/l lactate ratio is consistent with bacteria being the primary source. *Hum. Reprod.* 16: 1809–1813.

14 Colvin, C.W. and Abdullatif, H. (2013). Anatomy of female puberty: the clinical relevance of developmental changes in the reproductive system. *Clin. Anat.* 26: 115–129.

15 Gold, J.M. and Shrimanker, I. (2021, 2021). Physiology, vaginal. In: *StatPearls* [Internet]. Treasure Island (FL): StatPearls Publishing.

16 Nguyen, J.D. and Duong, H. (2021, 2022). Anatomy, Abdomen and Pelvis, Female External Genitalia. In: *StatPearls* [Internet]. Treasure Island (FL): StatPearls Publishing https://www.ncbi.nlm.nih.gov/books/NBK547703.

17 Sanchez, D.F. and Cubilla, A.L. (2022). Anatomy & histology-penis. http://PathologyOutlines.com website. https://www.pathologyoutlines.com/topic/penscrotumanat.html. Accessed January 9th, 2022.

18 Cold, C.J. and Taylor, J.R. (1999). The prepuce. *Br. J. Urol.* 83: 34–44.

19 Ganor, Y. and Bomsel, M. (2011). HIV-1 transmission in the male genital tract: HIV-1 entry at the foreskin. *Am. J. Reprod. Immunol.* 65 (3): 284–291. https://doi.org/10.1111/j.1600-0897.2010. 00933.x.

20 Sennepin, A., Real, F., Duvivier, M. et al. (2017). The human penis is a genuine immunological effector site. *Front. Immunol.* 8: 1732. https://doi.org/10.3389/fimmu.2017.01732.

21 Hickey, D.K., Patel, M.V., Fahey, J.V., and Wira, C.R. (2011). Innate and adaptive immunity at mucosal surfaces of the female reproductive tract: stratification and integration of immune protection against the transmission of sexually transmitted infections. *J. Reprod. Immunol.* 88 (2): 185–194. http://dx.doi.org/10.1016/j.jri.2011.01.005.

22 Pudney, J. and Anderson, D.J. (2010, 2011). Expression of toll-like receptors in genital tract tissues from normal and HIV-infected men: toll-like receptors in human male genital tissues. *Am. J. Reprod. Immunol.* 65 (1): 28–43. https://doi.org/10.1111/j.1600-0897 .2010. 00877.

7

Oral and Genital Microbiota

Vidya Pai[1] and S.R. Prabhu[2]

[1]*Department of Microbiology, Yenepoya Medical College, Mangaluru, India*
[2]*University of Queensland, School of Dentistry, Brisbane, Australia*

Introduction

Oral and genital mucosal surfaces make up complex mechanisms to provide the first-line defence against pathogens (see Chapter 6). They are colonised by a large number of bacteria, fungi and viruses that not only maintain a healthy orogenital environment but also influence the immune responses at these sites. Oral and genital mucosal surfaces are frequently involved in sexual contact between individuals. This may cause translocation of microorganisms from one site to the other during sexual activity. Normal microbial flora of the oral and genital sites has an important role to play in fighting against the sexually acquired pathogens. Understanding the basics of microbiota at these sites, therefore, is important for clinicians including dental professionals. A brief overview of the oral and genital microbiota is presented in this chapter.

Oral Microbiota

Oral Homeostasis

Mucosal immune responses in health and disease are defined by the equilibrium of host–microbial interactions [1]. The commensal microbial populations do not cause disease and may keep pathogenic species in check by not allowing them to adhere to mucosal surfaces. Colonisation of infant's mouth is associated with the mode of childbirth. In babies delivered vaginally, *Firmicutes* (the single largest group of bacteria), *Bacteroides* and *Actinobacteria* are most abundant, while *Bacteroides*, *Proteobacteria* and *Firmicutes* are most abundant in babies delivered by caesarean section [1]. The complexity of the developing oral microbiota increases particularly following tooth eruption. The microbial composition of the oral microbiota remains relatively stable over time, but, in older age, the carriage

Sexually Transmissible Oral Diseases, First Edition.
Edited by S.R. Prabhu, Nicholas van Wagoner, Jeff Hill and Shailendra Sawleshwarkar.
© 2023 John Wiley & Sons Ltd. Published 2023 by John Wiley & Sons Ltd.

of *Staphylococci* and *Enterobacteria* is more common. Yeasts are also more prevalent in the elderly [1].

Microbiota and Microbiome

Although terms such as microbiota and microbiome are used interchangeably, these two terms have subtle differences. Oral microbiota (oral microflora) refers to non-pathogenic microorganisms, such as bacteria, fungi and viruses, found within oral cavity. Oral microbiome is defined as the collective genome of microorganisms that reside in the oral cavity [2]. These are commensal organisms living in a symbiotic relationship, in which one organism lives near, on or within another organism and derives benefit thereof without injuring or helping the other.

Oral microbiota is the second largest microbial community in humans. The oral cavity has two types of surfaces on which bacteria can colonise: the hard and the soft tissues of teeth, and the oral mucosa, respectively [1, 2]. An ideal environment is provided by the oral cavity and associated nasopharyngeal regions for the growth of microorganisms. The normal temperature of the oral cavity on average is 37 °C without significant changes, which provides bacteria a stable environment to survive. Saliva also has a stable pH of 6.5–7, the favourable pH for most species of bacteria. It keeps the bacteria hydrated and serves as a medium for the transportation of nutrients to microorganisms [3]. Saliva washes these surfaces, which results in a monolayer of non-pathogenic microorganisms. The hard surfaces of the oral cavity are coated with a surplus of bacteria, known as biofilms, which are aggregates of a mixture of bacteria protected by the extracellular polysaccharide layer around them [3].

The oral microbiota contributes to oral and general well-being, and its loss can be detrimental to the health of the individual [4]. The complex equilibrium between resident species in the oral cavity is responsible for the maintenance of a healthy state (in symbiosis) or a state associated with disease (in dysbiosis) [4]. Modifiable factors driving oral dysbiosis include salivary gland dysfunction with changes in saliva flow and/or composition, poor oral hygiene, gingival inflammation and lifestyle choices, including dietary habits and smoking. The co-evolution to a harmonious coexistence is only valid as long as microbes remain in their natural habitat and are not disseminated to other body sites, where they can cause disease [4].

Resident bacteria have both pro- and anti-inflammatory activities that are crucial for maintaining homeostasis at heavily colonised sites such as the oral cavity [4, 5]. Immunomodulatory commensal bacteria are essential for maintaining healthy tissues, having multiple roles including priming immune responses to ensure rapid and efficient defences against pathogens. Commensal bacteria display pro-inflammatory and anti-inflammatory activities, and both are important in maintaining host–microbe homeostasis at heavily colonised sites [5]. Both saliva and gingival crevicular fluid (GCF) provide nutrients for microbial growth and contain components with antimicrobial activities. Saliva contains vital enzymes and proteins that help maintain a balanced microbiota. Many salivary components, including secretory immunoglobulin A, lactoferrin, lactoperoxidase, lysozyme, statherin and histatins, directly and indirectly regulate the microbiome, keeping it in balance [6].

Oral Commensal Population

It has been estimated that a minimum of 700 different species of microorganisms are present in the human oral cavity [7]. The gingival sulcus is the most-studied niche of microbial colonisation in the oral mucosa. The crevice between the hard surface of the teeth and the gingiva (gingival sulcus) harbours microbial communities that interact with the mucosal epithelial cells.

Bacteria

Of the commensal populations, bacteria are the main inhabitants of the oral cavity. In healthy mouths, these include *Streptococcus* spp., *Actinomyces* spp., *Veillonella* spp., *Fusobacteria, Porphyromonas* spp., *Prevotella* spp., *Treponemes, Nisseriae, Haemophilis* spp., *Eubacteria, Lactobacteria, Capnocytophaga* spp., *Eikenella* spp., *Leptotrichia, Peptostreptococci, Staphylococci* and *Propionibacterium* spp. [8]. Nutrition of oral bacteria is derived from starch and sucrose from the host diet; glycoprotein, minerals and vitamins from salivary sources; proteins from crevicular exudates, extracellular microbial products of the neighbouring bacteria and intracellular food storage granules [9].

Viruses

Viruses in the oral cavity are predominantly bacteriophages that live within bacteria, replicating and, eventually, destroying the bacterial cell. The exact role of viral communities in mouth is unclear; however, they may provide evolutionary advantages to their host bacteria [10].

Fungi

It has been estimated that about 85 species of fungi are present in the mouth with a predominance of *Candida* species. The most common commensal fungi and members of the basal oral mycobiome are the *Candida* genera. These are found in 70% of healthy individuals. Oral *Candida* species include *Candida tropicalis, Candida glabrata, Candida pseudotropicalis, Candida guillierimondii, Candida krusei, Candida lusitaniae, Candida parapsilosis* and *Candida stellatoidea*. The difference between commensalism and pathogenicity for *Candida albicans* seems to be the result of a fine balance between fungal virulence and host defence mechanisms [11]. The other genera of fungi like *Cladosporium, Aureobasidium, Saccharomycetales, Aspergillus, Fusarium* and *Cryptococcus* also are found to colonise the oral mucosal surfaces.

Other Organisms

Other commensal organisms include protozoa *Entamoeba gingivalis* and *Trichomonas tenax* [12].

The oral microbiota mediates microbial interspecies interactions and interacts with the oral cavity, thus creating a symbiotic relationship with the human host. Oral microbiota are important for the maturation and development of an appropriate oral immune response. The host immune system defends the host against pathogenic microbes and harmonise and protect commensal oral microbes [11, 12].

Female Genital Microbiota

The vaginal microbiota (VMB) is defined as a community of commensal, symbiotic and pathogenic microorganisms that colonise the vagina. The human vaginal mucosa has an abundant microflora. It is also exposed to spermatozoa and sexually transmitted pathogens. The mucosal environment in vagina frequently changes according to the cyclical hormonal changes in the female body. Menstrual cycle, pregnancy and menopause have major influence on the vaginal microflora. The vaginal commensal microflora is intricate and dynamic as it changes throughout the life of a female and acts as a mucosal defence against pathogens.

Common Microorganisms

Bacteria

Over 200 bacterial species are present in the vagina. Of these, more than 120 *Lactobacillus* species have been described. These comprise more than 70% of resident bacteria in women. The most common *Lactobacilllus* species include *Lactobacilllus acidophilus* and *Lactobacilllus fermentum* and less common are *Lactobacilllus plantarum, Lactobacilllus brevis, Lactobacilllus jensenii, Lactobacilllus casei, Lactobacilllus delbrueckii* and *Lactobacilllus salivarius.* Lactobacilli ferment glycogen to lactic acid and create an acidic environment that protects the vagina against opportunistic pathogens and vaginal infections. Lactobacilli dominance of VMB has been shown to guard the host from other opportunistic microbial infections, including bacteria such as *Neisseria gonorrhoeae* and *Chlamydia trachomatis,* and viruses such as human immunodeficiency virus (HIV) and human papilloma virus (HPV) and fungi (e.g. *C. albicans*). The lactic acid and antimicrobial compounds produced by Lactobacilli are hypothesised to underlie such protection [13].

Glycogen produced by vaginal epithelium (pubertal/premenopausal) is also responsible for symbiotic association between the host and vaginal Lactobacilli. The pH of the vagina is kept low (<4.5) and restricts the growth of many potential pathogens. They also produce hydrogen peroxide and contribute to the protection of the vaginal mucosa from potential pathogens. Healthy, normal VMB that is dominated by lactobacilli may differ among some ethnic groups [14]. Several studies have demonstrated that 7–33% of healthy asymptomatic women (especially Black and Hispanic) lack appreciable numbers of *Lactobacillus* species in the vagina. Instead, they have a VMB that consists of other lactic-acid-producing bacterial species such as *Atopobium* spp., *Leptospira* spp., *Leuconostoc* spp., *Megasphaera* spp., *Pediococci, Streptococci and Weissella species* [14]. *Staphylococcus* spp., *Streptococcus* spp., *Peptostreptococci, Bacteroides* spp., *Fusobacteria, Gardnerella vaginalis, Mobiluncus* spp., *Prevotella* spp., and Gram-negative enteric organisms *such as Escherichia coli, Mycoplasma* spp. *and Ureaplasma* spp. are the other bacterial species resident in the vagina. Before puberty, during pregnancy and post menopause, the pH of vagina is less acidic and hence vulnerable to infections. Occasionally yeasts (*Torulopsis* and *Candida* spp.) have been reported as vaginal flora in postmenopausal women [15].

It has been reported that the VMB is stable although a number of hosts and exogenous or behavioural factors, including sex hormones, pregnancy, ethnicity, condom use, male partner circumcision, menses, sexual activity, antibiotics, douching, lubricant use and smoking are likely to impact the cervicovaginal microbiota [16].

Opportunistic Fungi

Fungi

Though vastly outnumbered by its bacterial counterparts, fungi are important constituents of the vaginal ecosystem in many healthy women. *Candida* species are opportunistic fungal pathogens and common members of the human mycobiome. *C. albicans*, an opportunistic fungal pathogen, colonises 20% of women without causing any overt symptoms [17].

Abnormal vaginal flora may occur because of a sexually transmitted infection (STI) such as trichononiasis, colonisation by an organism which is not part of the normal vaginal community. Other microorganisms in this category include *Streptococcus pneumoniae, Haemophilus influenzae* or *Listeria monocytogenes*, or by overgrowth or increased virulence of an organism that is a constituent part of normal vaginal flora, e.g. *E. coli*. Alterations in vaginal flora do not necessarily imply disease or result in symptoms. Disease results from interplay between microbial virulence, numerical dominance, and the innate and adaptive immune response of the host [18].

Male Genital Microbiota

Information on the penile microbiota is remarkably deficient. Studies have used swabs from coronal sulcus and urine to determine the penile microbiota and the urethral microbiota respectively.

Common Microorganisms

The penile bacteria have aerobic, anaerobic, facultative anaerobic and microaerophilic profiles. Studies utilising swabs taken from the coronal sulcus demonstrate that the penile microbiota commonly contains bacteria similar to those found on the skin including *Corynebacteria* (diphtheroids) and *Staphylococcus* spp., as well as *Anerococcus* spp. Furthermore, the penile microbiota may contain anaerobic bacteria such as *Clostridia, Porphyromonas* spp. and *Prevotella* spp. [18]. Anatomy is also a major determinant of the genital microbiota in men, and the foreskin represents a unique physical and biochemical environment that harbours a specific microbiota different from that of the coronal sulcus. Removal of the foreskin during male circumcision causes dramatic changes in the male genital microbiota. Gram-negative communities disappear after circumcision [19]. Lactobacilli are not so prevalent in male genital tract. The possible transfer of penile flora into female partners leading to imbalance in vaginal flora further causing bacterial vaginosis is well documented [20].

References

1 Perez-Muñoz, M.E., Arrieta, M.-C., Ramer-Tait, A.E., and Walter, J. (2017). A critical assessment of the "sterile womb" and "in utero colonization" hypotheses: implications for research on the pioneer infant microbiome. *Microbiome* 5 (1): 48.

2 Zaura, E., Nicu, E.A., Krom, B.P., and Keijser, B.J. (2014). Acquiring and maintaining a normal oral microbiome: current perspective. *Front. Cell. Infect. Microbiol.* 4: 85. https://doi.org/10.3389/fcimb.2014.00085.

3 Lim, Y., Totsika, M., Morrison, M., and Punyadeera, C. (2017). Oral microbiome: a new biomarker reservoir for oral and oropharyngeal cancers. *Theranostics* 7: 4313–4321.

4 Kilian, M., Chapple, L.C., Hannig, M. et al. (2016). The oral microbiome – an update for oral healthcare professionals. *BDJ* 221 (10): 657–666.

5 Devine, D.A., March, P.D., and Josephine, M. (2015). Modulation of host response by oral commensal bacteria. *J. Oral Microbiol.* https://doi.org/10.3402/jom.v7.26941.

6 van't Hof, W., Veerman, E.C., Nieuw Amerongen, A.V., and Ligtenberg, A.J. (2014). Antimicrobial defense systems in saliva. *Monogr. Oral Sci.* 24: 40–51.

7 Park, Y.J. and Lee, H.K. (2018). The role of skin and orogenital microbiota in protective immunity and chronic immune-mediated inflammatory disease. *Front. Immunol.* 10: https://doi.org/10.3389/fimmu.2017.01955.

8 Arweiler, N.B. and Netuschil, L. (2016). The oral microbiota. *Adv. Exp. Med. Biol.* 902: 45–60. https://doi.org/10.1007/978-3-319-31248-4_4.

9 Avila, M., Ojcius, D.M., and Yilmaz, O. (2009). The oral microbiota: living with a permanent guest. *DNA Cell Biol.* 28: 405–411.

10 Halhoul, N. and Colvin, J.R. (1975). Virus-like particles in association with a microorganism from human gingival plaque. *Arch. Oral Biol.* 20: 833–836.

11 Kirchner, F.R., Littringer, K., Altmeier, S. et al. (2019). Persistence of *Candida albicans* in the oral mucosa induces a curbed inflammatory host response that is independent of immunosuppression. *Front. Immunol.* 10: 330.

12 Sharma, N., Bhatia, S., Sodhi, A.S., and Batra, N. (2018). Oral microbiome and health. *AIMS Microbiol.* 4: 42–66.

13 Wang, S., Wang, Q., Yang, E. et al. (2017). Antimicrobial compounds produced by vaginal *Lactobacillus crispatus* are able to strongly inhibit *Candida albicans* growth, hyphal formation and regulate virulence-related gene expressions. *Front. Microbiol.* 8: 564. https://doi.org/10.3389/fmicb.2017.00564.

14 Hearps, A.C., Tyssen, D., Srbinovski, D. et al. (2017). Vaginal lactic acid elicits an anti-inflammatory response from human cervicovaginal epithelial cells and inhibits production of pro-inflammatory mediators associated with HIV acquisition. *Mucosal Immunol.* 10 (6): 1480–1490. https://doi.org/10.1038/mi.2017.27.

15 Smith, B.C., Zolnik, C.P., Usyk, M. et al. (2016). Distinct ecological niche of anal, oral, and cervical mucosal microbiomes in adolescent women. *Yale J. Biol. Med.* 89 (3): 277–S 284.

16 Smith, S.B. and Ravel, J. (2017). The vaginal microbiota, host defence and reproductive physiology. *J. Physiol.* 595 (2): 451–463. https://doi.org/10.1113/JP271694.

17 Bradford, L.L. and Ravel, J. (2017). The vaginal mycobiome: a contemporary perspective on fungi in women's health and diseases. *Virulence* 8 (3): 342–351. https://doi.org/10.1080/21505594.2016.1237332.

18 Lamont, R.F., Sobel, J.D., Akins, R.A. et al. (2011). The vaginal microbiome: new information about genital tract flora using molecular based techniques. *BJOG* 118 (5): 533–549. https://doi.org/10.1111/j.1471-0528.2010.02840.x.

19 Harris, O., Anna Lise, W., Julia, P., and Tracy, L.M. (2020). The penile microbiota in uncircumcised and circumcised men: relationships with HIV and human papillomavirus infections and cervicovaginal microbiota. *Front. Med.* 7: 383. https://doi.org/10.3389/fmed.2020.00383.

20 Curtis, H., Dirk, G., Rob, K., and The Human Microbiome Project Consortium (2012). Structure, function and diversity of the healthy human microbiome. *Nature* 486: 207–214. https://doi.org/10.1038/nature11234.

8

Risky Sexual Behaviours

Vijayasarathi Ramanathan

Faculty of Medicine and Health, The University of Sydney, Sydney, Australia

Introduction

People engage in diverse sexual activities to experience and express their sexuality [1]. Risky sexual behaviour (RSB) is any activity that places an individual(s) at risk of, potential or actual, undesirable outcomes (e.g. contracting sexually transmitted infections [STIs], human immunodeficiency virus [HIV] or unwanted pregnancy). RSB substantially contributes to disease burden [2]. RSBs are reported based on the specific sex act (e.g. condomless penovaginal/penoanal intercourse, unprotected oral–anogenital contact). RSB is also used to describe people who are considered 'at risk/high risk' based on their sexual behaviours (e.g. unprotected sex with multiple partners, sexual debut at a young age [3] or sex under the influence of alcohol/substance) [4]; people engaged in (unregulated) commercial sex work [5]; sex with a partner(s) who injects or has ever injected drugs; or sex with a high-risk partner [6].

Challenges with Defining RSB

There is no standardised definition for RSB because the way 'risk' is operationalised tends to vary depending on the concerned sexual behaviour and the target/study population. Multiple factors [4, 7, 8] have been used in attempts to operationalise RSB – the sex act (e.g. anal intercourse); non-engagement and/or inconsistency in risk mitigation (e.g. condom or contraceptive); the number of sexual partners; associated non-sexual behaviours that increase the likelihood of sexual activity (e.g. sex under the influence of alcohol/substance); relational nature of the persons involved (e.g. within or outside of a steady relationship); the context in which the act of sex takes place (e.g. coercion); and the impact of online

Sexually Transmissible Oral Diseases, First Edition.
Edited by S.R. Prabhu, Nicholas van Wagoner, Jeff Hill and Shailendra Sawleshwarkar.
© 2023 John Wiley & Sons Ltd. Published 2023 by John Wiley & Sons Ltd.

Table 8.1 Definitions of risky sexual behaviour.

Author	Definition
Strunin et al.	Sexual behaviour as a behaviour that increases likelihood of contracting sexually transmitted infections
Dublin et al.	Anal/oral sexual intercourse or vaginal intercourse without condom or other contraception
Cooper	Having multiple/casual partners, not using condom during sexual intercourse, having intercourse under influence of alcohol
IIPS (NFHS-3)	Sexual intercourse, within last 12 months, with someone who is neither a spouse nor a cohabiting partner
Kumari and Nair	Sexual intercourse with two or more partners with improper or inconsistent condom use and sexual relations of unmarried people in an exclusive relationship
Imaledo et al.	Early age of sexual debut, premarital sex without protection, sex in exchange of gifts
Chikovani et al.	Occasional or paid sexual partners, unprotected sexual intercourse.
Chanakira et al.	Sexual behaviour which increases the chances of sexual diseases and sometimes unwanted pregnancy
Ritchwood et al.	Unprotected intercourse, having multiple sexual partners, and having intercourse with an intravenous drug user (IVDU)
Mirzaei et al.	Sexual behaviour that increases the chance of a negative outcome. Negative consequences have been defined in the form of family conflicts, damage to relationships, legal disputes or financial problems.
CDC	Sexual intercourse with multiple partners, without using condom, under the influence of drugs, alcohol or being forced to have sex. These behaviours place them at risk of contracting sexually transmitted diseases, HIV or unintended pregnancy

Source: Chawla and Sarkar [7] / SAGE Publications.

social networking to find casual and/or anonymous sex partners [9]. Some of the definitions of RSB, as shown in Table 8.1 [7], are highly specific and prescriptive while others are broad and inclusive.

The Triad of RSB

RSB is a complex phenomenon that encompasses three individual, but overlapping, dimensions – human behaviour, sexual pleasure and voluntary risk taking (Figure 8.1). Human behaviour is the way a person 'acts' in response to internal (thoughts and feelings) and/or external (environmental including other people) stimuli and serves two distinct purposes: communication and function (survival, recreational, transactional and relational) [10]. Sexual pleasure is recognised as 'the physical and/or psychological satisfaction and enjoyment derived from shared or solitary erotic experiences, including thoughts, fantasies, dreams, emotions and feelings' [11]. Voluntary risk taking is defined as 'an activity, in

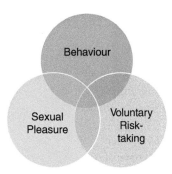

Figure 8.1 Triad of risky sexual behaviour.

which individuals engage, is perceived by them to be in some sense risky but is undertaken deliberately and from choice' [12]. All three dimensions of RSB are subjected to influence by several factors – biomedical, psycho-socio-cultural and interpersonal.

Conceptual Frameworks of RSB

It is a challenge to assess and risk stratify a specific sexual act due to the fluid nature of sexual behaviours and difficulty in eliciting an accurate sexual history. Not all who engage in RSB are misinformed or ignorant of the risks involved. This raises some very important questions about the person who voluntarily engages in an RSB. Why does this person engage in RSB despite knowing the (negative) consequence(s)? What goes through the mind of this person during the 'heat of the moment' (e.g. deciding to take off the condom half-way through sexual intercourse)? No one theory/model precisely explains why some people always engage in RSB while others not, and why some people decide to take risk at some, but not all, sexual encounters. One such theory and one model are briefly mentioned in the following section to help create a framework to duly understand and address RSB in a clinical or community setting.

The theory of planned behaviour (TPB) [1] postulates that an individual's intention to behave in a specific way (e.g. whether to use condom or not) depends on that person's attitude towards that behaviour (e.g. condoms would diminish the pleasure), the subject norm (e.g. my friends have never used condoms and had no issues) and perceived behaviour control (e.g. putting on a condom at the peak of sexual arousal is difficult). The TPB highlights that the intention to act is the single best predictor of a specific behaviour under volitional control (e.g. using condoms). A recent study found the constructs of the TPB to be highly predictive of safer sex behavioural patterns among substance users [13].

The dual control model [14] postulates that whether sexual response and associated arousal occur in a particular individual, in a particular situation, is ultimately determined by the balance between two neurobiological systems: the sexual activation or excitation system and the sexual inhibition system. The model recognises that individuals vary in their propensity for both sexual excitation and inhibition (related to performance and/or consequence). Individuals with an unusually high propensity for excitation and/or low propensity for inhibition would be more likely to engage in RSB or problematic sexual behaviour.

Oral Sexual Behaviour, Oral Health and STIs

Oral sex, often referred as oro-genital sex or oro-anal sex is a form of sexual stimulation using the mouth, lips or tongue. Oral sex involves fellatio oral–penis contact by licking and sucking, cunnilingus (oral–vaginal contact that includes the vagina and the vulva) or anilingus (oral–anus stimulation using the tongue or lips). In a broader context, oral sex could also mean deep kissing (aka French kissing), which does not involve the genitalia. The Global Survey of Sexual Attitudes and Behaviours that surveyed 27 500 men and women in 29 countries reported a high prevalence of oral (both giving and receiving) sex amongst all groups (heterosexual, homosexual and bisexual men and women) [15]. Oral–genital sex is commonly practised amongst youth with up to 1 in 2 adolescents reporting oral–genital sex prior to any other form of sexual intercourse and likely represents the generally held belief that oral sex is a safer alternative to other types of penetrative (peno-anal or peno-vaginal) sex [16]. While the risks associated with oral sex are quite low, pre-ejaculatory fluid, semen, vaginal secretions, menstrual blood, broken mucosal lining or bleeding gums (gingivitis or periodontitis), dental carious lesions and active sores could facilitate transmission of STI, especially viral STIs [17–20].

This chapter has provided some basic information and insight about sexual behaviours in general and more so about the RSB from a dental clinician's perspective. Oral sex, even though the risk is low, is well considered as a mode of transmission of STIs. Societal attitude that oral sex is 'risk-free', in comparison to other forms of RSB makes it highly challenging to promote the use of condoms or dental dams for oral–genital sex. Our understanding of the pathology, epidemiology and medical management of different STIs (including HIV) has certainly advanced over many decades. On the other hand, advancement in critical understanding and addressing (risky) sexual behaviours has been slower and poses a challenge for scientific enquiry [2]. Acknowledging the complexity of RSB, eliciting a thorough biopsychosexual history, and duly addressing the factors associated with RSB are essential to have effective risk reduction strategies for STIs within an oral health clinical setting and to promote safe sex practices at a public health level.

Sexually transmitted disease risk and oral sex are further discussed in Chapter 9.

References

1 Brown, J.L. (2013). Sexual Behavior. In: *Encyclopedia of Behavioral Medicine* (ed. M.D. Gellman and J.R. Turner), 1773–1774. New York: Springer https://doi.org/10.1007/978-1-4419-1005-9_667.

2 Wellings, K., Collumbien, M., Slaymaker, E. et al. (2006). Sexual behaviour in context: a global perspective. *The Lancet (British edition)* 368 (9548): 1706–1728. https://doi.org/10.1016/S0140-6736(06)69479-8.

3 Kebede, A., Molla, B., and Gerensea, H. (2018). Assessment of risky sexual behavior and practice among Aksum University students, Shire Campus, Shire Town, Tigray, Ethiopia, 2017. *BMC. Res. Notes* 11 (1): 88. https://doi.org/10.1186/s13104-018-3199-7.

4 Chanakira, E., O'Cathain, A., Goyder, E.C., and Freeman, J.V. (2014). Factors perceived to influence risky sexual behaviours among university students in the United Kingdom: a qualitative telephone interview study. *BMC Public Health* 14 (1): 1055. https://doi.org/10.1186/1471-2458-14-1055.

5 Spice, W. (2007). Management of sex workers and other high-risk groups. *Occup. Med.* 57 (5): 322–328. https://doi.org/10.1093/occmed/kqm045.

6 Stoner, B.P., Whittington, W.L.H., Aral, S.O. et al. (2003). Avoiding risky sex partners: perception of partners' risks *v* partners' self reported risks. *Sex. Transm. Infect.* 79 (3): 197–201. https://doi.org/10.1136/sti.79.3.197.

7 Chawla, N. and Sarkar, S. (2019). Defining "High-risk Sexual Behavior" in the context of substance use. *J. Psychosexual Health* 1 (1): 26–31. https://doi.org/10.1177/263183181 8822015.

8 Gupta, G.R., Parkhurst, J.O., Ogden, J.A. et al. (2008). Structural approaches to HIV prevention. *Lancet* 372 (9640): 764–775. https://doi.org/10.1016/s0140-6736(08)60887-9.

9 Holloway, I.W., Dunlap, S., Del Pino, H.E. et al. (2014). Online social networking, sexual risk and protective behaviors: considerations for clinicians and researchers. *Curr. Addict. Rep.* 1 (3): 220–228. https://doi.org/10.1007/s40429-014-0029-4.

10 NSW Health (2020). What is Behaviour? https://doi.org/10.1016/S0140-6736(06)69479-8.

11 World Association for Sexual Health (2019). Declaration on Sexual Pleasure. https://worldsexualhealth.net/declaration-on-sexual-pleasure/

12 Zinn, J.O. (2019). The meaning of risk-taking – key concepts and dimensions. *J. Risk Res.* 22 (1): 1–15. https://doi.org/10.1080/13669877.2017.1351465.

13 Khani Jeihooni, A., Kouhpayeh, A., Najafi, S., and Bazrafshan, M.-R. (2019). Application theory of planned behavior on promotion of safe sexual behaviors among drug users. *J. Subst. Abus.* 24 (3): 293–299. https://doi.org/10.1080/14659891.2018.1562575.

14 Bancroft, J., Graham, C.A., Janssen, E., and Sanders, S.A. (2009). The dual control model: current status and future directions. *J. Sex Res.* 46 (2–3): 121–142. https://doi.org/10.1080/00224490902747222.

15 Kevan, W. (2009). A global survey of sexual behaviours. *J. Family Reprod. Health* 3 (2): 39.

16 Saini, R., Saini, S., and Sharma, S. (2010). Oral sex, oral health and orogenital infections. *J. Glob. Infect.* 2 (1): 57–62. https://doi.org/10.4103/0974-777X.59252.

17 Limeres Posse, J., Diz Dios, P., and Scully, C. (2017). Viral diseases transmissible by kissing. *Saliva Prot. Transm. Dis.* 53–92: https://doi.org/10.1016/B978-0-12-813681-2.00004-4.

18 Glynn, T.R., Operario, D., Montgomery, M. et al. (2017). The duality of oral sex for men who have sex with men: an examination into the increase of sexually transmitted infections amid the age of HIV prevention. *AIDS Patient Care STDS* 31 (6): 261–267.

19 Turek, E.M., Fairley, C.K., Tabesh, M. et al. (2020). HIV, sexually transmitted infections and sexual practices among male sex workers attending a sexual health clinic in Melbourne, Australia, 2010–2018. *Sex. Transm. Dis.* 48 (2): 103–108.

20 Drake, V.E., Fakhry, C., Windon, M.J. et al. (2021). Timing, number, and type of sexual partners associated with risk of oropharyngeal cancer. *Cancer* 127 (7): 1029–1038.

9

Sexually Transmitted Disease Risk and Oral Sex

CDC, Division of STD Prevention, National Center for HIV, Viral Hepatitis, STD, and TB Prevention, Atlanta, GA, USA (https://www.cdc.gov/std/healthcomm/ stdfactstdriskandoralsex.htm) CDC Fact sheet.

Introduction

Many sexually transmitted diseases (STDs) can be spread through oral sex. Using a condom, dental dam or other barrier method every time the person has oral sex can reduce the risk of giving or getting an STD. There is little to no risk of getting or transmitting HIV from oral sex.

What Is Oral Sex?

Oral sex involves using the mouth, lips or tongue to stimulate the penis (fellatio), vagina (cunnilingus) or anus (anilingus) of a sex partner. The penis and testicles and the vagina and area around the vagina are also called the genitals or genital areas.

How Common Is Oral Sex?

Oral sex is commonly practiced by sexually active adults. More than 85% of sexually active adults aged 18–44 years reported having had oral sex at least once with a partner of the opposite sex. A separate survey conducted during 2011–2015 found that 41% of teenagers aged 15–19 years reported having had oral sex with a partner of the opposite sex.

Many STDs, as well as other infections, can be spread through oral sex. Anyone exposed to an infected partner can get an STD in the mouth, throat, genitals or rectum. The risk of getting an STD from oral sex, or spreading an STD to others through oral sex, depends on several things, including the particular STD, the sex acts practiced, how common the STD is in the population to which the sex partners belong and the number of specific sex acts performed.

In general, it may be possible to get some STDs in the mouth or throat from giving oral sex to a partner with a genital or anal/rectal infection, particularly from giving oral sex to a

Sexually Transmissible Oral Diseases, First Edition.
Edited by S.R. Prabhu, Nicholas van Wagoner, Jeff Hill and Shailendra Sawleshwarkar.
© 2023 John Wiley & Sons Ltd. Published 2023 by John Wiley & Sons Ltd.

partner with an infected penis. It also may be possible to get certain STDs on the penis (and possibly the vagina, anus or rectum) from getting oral sex from a partner with a mouth or throat infection. It is possible to have an STD in more than one area at the same time, for example in the throat and the genitals. Several STDs that may be transmitted by oral sex can then spread throughout the body (i.e. syphilis, gonorrhoea and intestinal infections).

Anilingus (or oral sex involving the anus) can transmit hepatitis A and B, intestinal parasites like *Giardia*, and bacteria like *Escherichia coli* and *Shigella*. STDs can be spread to a sex partner even when the infected partner has no signs or symptoms. If you are infected with an STD, you might not know it because many STDs may have no symptoms.

Which STDs Can be Passed on from Oral Sex?

- *Chlamydia trachomatis*
- Gonorrhoea
- Syphilis
- Herpes
- Human papillomavirus (HPV) infections
- Human immune virus deficiency virus infections (HIV)

Chlamydia (*C. Trichomoniasis*): Risk of Infection from Oral Sex

- Giving oral sex to a partner with an infected penis can result in getting chlamydia in the throat.
- Giving oral sex to a partner with an infected vagina or urinary tract may result in getting chlamydia in the throat.*
- Giving oral sex to a partner with an infected rectum might result in getting chlamydia in the throat.*
- Getting oral sex on the penis from a partner with chlamydia in the throat can result in getting chlamydia of the penis.
- Getting oral sex on the vagina from a partner with chlamydia in the throat might result in getting chlamydia of the vagina or urinary tract.*
- Getting oral sex on the anus from a partner with chlamydia in the throat might result in getting chlamydia in the rectum.*

(Statements followed by an asterisk (*) have not been well studied.)
Areas of initial infection include throat, genitals, urinary tract and rectum.

Gonorrhoea: Risk of Infection from Oral Sex

- Giving oral sex to a partner with an infected penis can result in getting gonorrhoea in the throat.
- Giving oral sex to a partner with an infected vagina or urinary tract might result in getting gonorrhoea in the throat.*
- Giving oral sex to a partner with an infected rectum might result in getting gonorrhoea in the throat.*

- Getting oral sex on the penis from a partner with gonorrhoea in the throat may result in getting gonorrhoea of the penis.
- Getting oral sex on the vagina from a partner with gonorrhoea in the throat might result in getting gonorrhoea of the vagina or urinary tract.*
- Getting oral sex on the anus from a partner with gonorrhoea in the throat might result in getting gonorrhoea in the rectum.*

(Statements followed by an asterisk (*) have not been well studied.)
Areas of initial infection include throat, genitals, urinary tract and rectum.

Syphilis: Risk of Infection from Oral Sex

- Giving oral sex to a partner with a syphilis sore or rash on the genitals or anus can result in getting syphilis.
- Getting oral sex from a partner with a syphilis sore or rash on the lips or mouth, or in the throat, can result in getting syphilis.
- Another important factor that affects the risk of spreading syphilis is how long an infected partner has had syphilis.

Areas of initial infection include lips, mouth, throat, genitals, anus and rectum.

Herpes: Risk of Infection from Oral Sex

- Giving oral sex to a partner with herpes on the genital area, anus, buttocks or in the rectum may result in getting herpes on the lips, mouth or in the throat.
- Getting oral sex from a partner with herpes on the lips, mouth or in the throat can result in getting herpes on the genital area, anus, buttocks or in the rectum.

Areas of initial infection include lips, mouth, throat, genital area, anus, rectum and buttocks.

HIV Infection: Risk of Infection from Oral Sex

- Giving oral sex on the penis of a partner with HIV can result in getting HIV. The risk of infection is lower than the risks from vaginal or anal sex.
- Giving oral sex on the vagina of a partner with HIV may result in getting HIV. The risk of infection is thought to be very low.
- Giving oral sex on the anus of a partner with HIV may result in getting HIV. There are a few reports of transmission from this type of oral sex.
- Getting oral sex on the penis from a partner with HIV may result in getting HIV. This risk is thought to be very low and has not been well studied. Getting oral sex on the vagina from a partner with HIV might result in getting HIV. This risk is thought to be extremely low and has not been well studied.
- Getting oral sex on the anus from a partner with HIV might result in getting HIV. There are a few reports of transmission from this type of oral sex.
- Another important factor that affects the risk of HIV spread is the virus level (i.e. viral load) in an infected partner's blood and other body fluids at the time of the sexual

encounter. An undetectable HIV viral load eliminates the risk of spreading HIV from oral sex.

Current literature identifies the risk of HIV transmission through oral sex as less of a risk than that of unprotected receptive penile–anal sexual exposure (0.1–3%) or receptive penile–vaginal exposure (0.1–0.2%). While saliva inhibits HIV infectivity and has been shown to kill up to 90% of HIV-infected cells and break apart HIV into non-infectious components. If HIV cells remain present, there is a theoretical possibility of transmission from the cells to the oral mucosa due to flossing and/or any other trauma to the oral mucosa. Additionally, the Centres for Disease Control and Prevention outline several co-factors that may increase the risk of HIV transmission as a result of oral sex, including bleeding gums.

HPV Infection: Risk of Infection from Oral Sex

- Giving oral sex to a partner with an HPV-infected penis or genital area can result in getting HPV in the throat.
- Giving oral sex to a partner with an HPV-infected vagina or genital area can result in getting HPV in the throat.
- Giving oral sex to a partner with HPV on the anus or in the rectum may result in getting HPV in the throat.*
- Getting oral sex from a partner with HPV in the throat might result in getting HPV on the genital area, anus or rectum.*

(Statements followed by an asterisk (*) have not been well studied.)

Areas of infection include mouth, throat, genital area, vagina, cervix, anus and rectum.

HPV vaccine protects against transmission of certain types of HPV. It is recommended for all boys and girls at ages 11–12, as well as for everyone through age 26 if not vaccinated already.

Is Oral Sex Safer than Vaginal or Anal Sex?

- Many STDs can be spread through oral sex. However, it is difficult to compare the exact risks of getting specific STDs from specific types of sexual activity. This is partly because most people who have oral sex also have vaginal or anal sex. Also, a few studies have looked at the risks of getting STDs other than HIV from giving oral sex on the vagina or anus, compared to giving oral sex on the penis.
- Studies have shown that the risk of getting HIV from having oral sex with an infected partner (either giving or getting oral sex) is much lower than the risk of getting HIV from anal or vaginal sex with an infected partner. This may not be true for other STDs – in one study of gay men with syphilis, one out of five reported having only oral sex. Getting HIV from oral sex may be extremely low, but it is hard to know the exact risk. If you are having oral sex, you should still protect yourself. Repeated unprotected oral sex exposure to HIV may represent a considerable risk for spread of other STDs for which the risk of spread through oral sex has not been as well studied.
- It is possible that getting certain STDs, such as chlamydia or gonorrhoea, in the throat may not pose as a great threat to an infected person's health as getting an STD in the genital area or rectum.

o Having these infections in the throat might increase the risk of getting HIV. Having gonorrhoea in the throat also may lead to spread of the disease throughout the body. In addition, having infections of chlamydia and gonorrhoea in the throat may make it easier to spread these infections to others through oral sex. This is especially important for gonorrhoea, since throat infections can be harder to treat than urinary, genital or rectal infections.

o Infections from certain STDs, such as syphilis and HIV, spread throughout the body. Therefore, infections that are acquired in the throat may lead to the same health problems as infections acquired in the genitals or rectum.

o Mouth and throat infections by certain types of HPV may develop into oral or neck cancer.

What May Increase the Chances of Giving or Getting an STD through Oral Sex?

It is possible that certain factors may increase a person's chances of getting HIV or other STDs during oral sex if exposed to an infected partner, such as

- having poor oral health, which can include tooth decay, gum disease or bleeding gums, and oral cancer
- having sores in the mouth or on the genitals
- being exposed to the 'pre-cum' or 'cum' (also known as pre-ejaculate or ejaculate) of an infected partner

However, no scientific studies have been done to show whether or not these factors actually do increase the risk of getting HIV or STDs from oral sex.

What Can Be Done to Prevent STD Transmission during Oral Sex?

- Chances of giving or getting STDs during oral sex can be lowered by using a condom, dental dam or other barrier method every time when oral sex is performed.
- The only way to avoid STDs is to not have vaginal, anal or oral sex. For sexually active individuals, the following things may lower their chances of getting STDs
- Being in a long-term mutually monogamous relationship with a partner who is not infected with an STD (e.g. a partner who has been tested and has negative STD test results) and using latex condoms the right way every time during sex.
- It is important to remember that many infected individuals may be unaware of their infection because STDs often have no symptoms and are unrecognised.
- Sexually active individuals should get tested regularly for STDs and HIV and talk to their partner(s) about STDs.
- If an STD is suspected, sexual activity should be stopped, and the individual should get tested.

• It is important to talk openly with the healthcare provider about any activities including oral sex that might put the individual at risk for an STD.

Acknowledgement:

This Fact Sheet has been reproduced with permission from the CDC.

Recommended Readings

Patel, P., Borkowf, C.B., Brooks, J.T. et al. (2014). Estimating per-act HIV transmission risk: a systematic review. *AIDS* 28 (10): 1509–1519.

Habel, M.A., Leichliter, J.S., Dittus, P.J. et al. (2018). Heterosexual anal and oral sex in adolescents and adults in the United States, 2011–2015. *Sex. Transm. Dis.* 45 (12): 775–782.

Sparling, P.F., Swartz, M.N., Musher, D.M., and Healy, B.P. (2008). Clinical manifestations of syphilis. In: *Sexually Transmitted Diseases*, 4e (ed. K.K. Holmes, P.F. Sparling, W.E. Stamm, et al.), 662–684. New York: McGraw-Hill.

Centers for Disease Control and Prevention. Questions and answers on the use of HIV medications to help prevent the transmission of HIV. 4-13-2010. 2-7-2012.

Jones, R.B., Rabinovitch, R.A., Katz, B.P. et al. (1985). Chlamydia trachomatis in the pharynx and rectum of heterosexual patients at risk for genital infection. *Ann. Internal Med.* 102: 757–762.

Templeton, D.J., Jin, F., Imrie, J. et al. (2008). Prevalence, incidence, and risk factors for pharyngeal chlamydia in the community-based health in men (HIM) cohort of homosexual men in Sydney, Australia. *Sex. Transm. Infect.* 84: 361–363.

Benn, P.D., Rooney, G., Carder, C. et al. (2007). *Chlamydia trachomatis* and *Neisseria gonorrhoeae* infection and the sexual behaviour of men who have sex with men. *Sex. Transm. Infect.* 83: 106–112.

Bernstein, K.T., Stephens, S.C., Barry, P.M. et al. (2009). *Chlamydia trachomatis* and *Neisseria gonorrhoeae* transmission from the oropharynx to the urethra among men who have sex with men. *Clin. Infect. Dis.* 49: 1793–1797.

Centers for Disease Control and Prevention (2010). Sexually transimitted diseases treatment guidelines, 2010. *Morbidity Mortality Wkly. Rep.* 59: 1–110.

World Health Organization. Consultation on STD interventions for preventing HIV: what is the evidence? 1–54. 2000. UNAIDS/00.06E, WHO/HIS/2000.02. 2-19-2010.

Murray, A.B., Greenhouse, P.R., Nelson, W.L. et al. (1991). Coincident acquisition of Neisseria gonorrhoeae and HIV from fellatio. *Lancet* 338: 830.

Wong, M.L. and Chan, R.K. (1999). A prospective study of pharyngeal gonorrhoea and inconsistent condom use for oral sex among female brothel-based sex workers in Singapore. *Int. J. STD & AIDS* 10: 595–599.

Morris, S.R., Klausner, J.D., Buchbinder, S.P. et al. (2006). Prevalence and incidence of pharyngeal gonorrhea in a longitudinal sample of men who have sex with men: the EXPLORE study. *Clin. Infect. Dis.* 43: 1284–1289.

Wong, M.L., Chan, R.K., and Koh, D. (2002). Promoting condoms for oral sex: impact on pharyngeal gonorrhea among female brothel-based sex workers. *Sex. Transm. Dis.* 29: 311–318.

Jin, F., Prestage, G.P., Imrie, J. et al. (2010). Anal sexually transmitted infections and risk of HIV infection in homosexual men. *J. Acquired Immune Deficiency Syndromes JAIDS* 53: 144–149.

Peterman, T.A. and Furness, B.W. (2007). The resurgence of syphilis among men who have sex with men. [Review] [65 refs]. *Curr. Opin. Infect. Dis.* 20: 54–59.

Centers for Disease Control and Prevention (CDC) (2004). Transmission of primary and secondary syphilis by oral sex–Chicago, Illinois, 1998–2002. *MMWR Morbidity & Mortality Wkly. Report* 53: 966–968.

Campos-Outcalt, D. and Hurwitz, S. (2002). Female-to-female transmission of syphilis: a case report. *Sex. Transm. Dis.* 29: 119–120.

McCall, M.B., van Lith-Verhoeven, J.J., van Crevel, R. et al. (2004). Ocular syphilis acquired through oral sex in two HIV-infected patients. *Netherlands J. Med.* 62: 206–208.

Lafferty, W.E., Coombs, R.W., Benedetti, J. et al. (1987). Recurrences after oral and genital herpes simplex virus infection. Influence of site of infection and viral type. *N. Engl. J. Med.* 316: 1444–1449.

Smith, E.M., Ritchie, J.M., Summersgill, K.F. et al. (2004). Age, sexual behavior and human papillomavirus infection in oral cavity and oropharyngeal cancers. *Int. J. Cancer* 108: 766–772.

D'Souza, G., Kreimer, A.R., Viscidi, R. et al. (2007). Case-control study of human papillomavirus and oropharyngeal cancer. *N. Engl. J. Med.* 356: 1944–1956.

D'Souza, G., Agrawal, Y., Halpern, J. et al. (2009). Oral sexual behaviors associated with prevalent oral human papillomavirus infection. *J. Infect. Dis.* 199: 1263–1269.

Castro, T.P. and Bussoloti, F. (2006). I. Prevalence of human papillomavirus (HPV) in oral cavity and oropharynx. [Review] [82 refs]. *Revista Brasileira de Otorrinolaringologia* 72: 272–282.

Terai, M., Hashimoto, K., Yoda, K., and Sata, T. (1999). High prevalence of human papillomaviruses in the normal oral cavity of adults. *Oral Microbiol. Immunol.* 14: 201–205.

Gillison, M.L. (2008). Human papillomavirus-related diseases: oropharynx cancers and potential implications for adolescent HPV vaccination. *J Adolesc Health* 43(4 Suppl): S52–S60. https://doi.org/10.1016/j.jadohealth.2008.07.002.

Keet, I.P., van brecht, L.N., Sandfort, T.G. et al. (1992). Orogenital sex and the transmission of HIV among homosexual men. *AIDS* 6: 223–226.

del Romero, J., Marincovich, B., Castilla, J. et al. (2002). Evaluating the risk of HIV transmission through unprotected orogenital sex. *AIDS* 16: 1296–1297.

Page-Shafer, K., Shiboski, C.H., Osmond, D.H. et al. (2002). Risk of HIV infection attributable to oral sex among men who have sex with men and in the population of men who have sex with men. *AIDS* 16: 2350–2352.

Baggaley, R.F., White, R.G., and Boily, M.C. (2008). Systematic review of orogenital HIV-1 transmission probabilities. [Review] [29 refs]. *Int. J. Epidemiol.* 37: 1255–1265.

Bratt, G.A., Berglund, T., Glantzberg, B.L. et al. (1997). Two cases of oral-to-genital HIV-1 transmission. *Int. J. STD & AIDS* 8: 522–525.

Edwards, S. and Carne, C. (1998). Oral sex and the transmission of viral STIs. [Review] [99 refs]. *Sex. Transm. Infect.* 74: 6–10.

Weinstock, H. and Workowski, K.A. (2009). Pharyngeal gonorrhea: an important reservoir of infection? *Clin. Infect. Dis.* 49: 1798–1800.

Robinson, E.K. and Evans, B.G. (1999). Oral sex and HIV transmission. [Review] [16 refs]. *AIDS* 13: 737–738.

Hawkins, D.A. (2001). Oral sex and HIV transmission. *Sex. Transm. Infect.* 77: 307–308.

Section 3

Oral Manifestations of Sexually Transmissible Diseases

10

Oral Traumatic Lesions Associated with Oral Sex
S.R. Prabhu

University of Queensland, School of Dentistry, Brisbane, Australia

Introduction

Oral sex is a common sexual practice between both heterosexual and same-sex couples [1]. Couples of all sexual orientations may engage in oral sex before sexual intercourse, during or after intercourse [1–5]. Non-coital sexual activities including oral sex are common among adolescents [1]. Reports indicate that more than 85% of sexually active adults aged 18 to 44 years had oral sex at least once with a partner of the opposite sex [1] and 41% of teenagers aged 15 to 19 years had oral sex with a partner of the opposite sex. Between 14% and 50% of adolescents have had oral sex before their first experience with sexual intercourse [1–3, 5]. Reports also indicate that a significant number of adolescents had more oral sex than vaginal sex and that a few adolescents who engage in oral sex use barrier protection [1, 6, 7].

Many sexually transmitted infections (STIs), as well as other infections, can be spread through oral sex [1–4, 6–8]. Anyone exposed to an infected partner can get an STD in the mouth, throat, genitals or rectum. The risk of getting an STD from oral sex, or spreading an STD to others through oral sex, depends on several things, including the particular STD, the sex acts practiced, how common the STD is in the population to which the sex partners belong and the number of specific sex acts performed [1–4, 6–8].

Oral Sex and Traumatic Oral Lesions

The risk of contracting sexually transmitted infections associated with oral sex has received much attention. However, the risk of oral traumatic lesions associated with oral sex appears to have received less attention because of their common asymptomatic nature. When the lesions are symptomatic, the patient may not be aware of its cause. Even when the patient is aware of the cause of oral lesions, the clinician may not be able to obtain the history of oral sex.

Sexually Transmissible Oral Diseases, First Edition.
Edited by S.R. Prabhu, Nicholas van Wagoner, Jeff Hill and Shailendra Sawleshwarkar.

A few cases of traumatic lesions caused by oral sex have been published in the medical [9–13] and dental [14–17] literature. Palatal lesions secondary to fellatio have been reported in the age group of 18–59 years, but predominantly in young women in their early 20s [14, 16]. Oral lesions have also been reported in young children, often around the age of 3 years, secondary to sexual abuse [15, 18]. Estimates of mucosal lesions associated with cunnilingus are not available.

Clinical Features of Fellatio Associated Oral Lesions

Fellatio has become popular, particularly among young people. The contact of the palate with the penile glans creates negative pressure while sucking. Fellatio-associated traumatic blood vessel injuries of the palate have been reported as palatal ecchymoses, palatal erythema, palatal haemorrhage, palatal petechiae and palatal purpura [9, 13, 15, 19, 20]. Fellatio may cause dilatation of the palatal blood vessels due to blunt trauma and result in haematoma. The pathogenesis of fellatio-associated palatal haemorrhagic lesions is multifactorial. Direct and forceful contact of the distal penis against the palate may result in mucosal injury with the rupture of submucosal vessels and haemorrhage, or it may be secondary to an intense reflex palato-pharyngeal spasm brought on during fellatio. The concurrent negative pressure created through irrumation: (the penetration of a mouth with a penis) has a major contributory role in the mechanism of injury. Occasionally these lesions may be associated with secondary candidal infections [9, 13, 15, 19, 20].

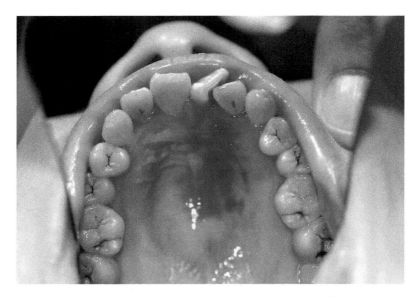

Figure 10.1 Erythema of the palate due to fellatio. Source: Muthu et al. [13]. Reproduced with permission from Scientific Scholar.

The palatal traumatic lesions may be asymptomatic and remain unnoticed. Fellatio-associated palatal purpura usually appears on the soft palate and spares the uvula but can also develop at the junction of the hard and soft palates and infrequently on the hard palate [12, 14, 19–21] (Figure 10.1). Although submucosal haemorrhages are usually asymptomatic, they may be discovered during tooth brushing, flossing or inspection of the oral cavity. Many people may not initially associate palatal lesions with oral sex. In addition to petechiae and purpura, fellatio-associated submucosal trauma can show erythematous lesions, papules, vesicles, erosions and/or ulcers [12, 14, 19–22]. The lesions usually appear in the midline of the palate but may become large enough to involve both sides of the palate. Biopsy and histopathologic assessment of the lesions are not required for diagnosis, unless other causes of palatal trauma are suspected [12, 14, 19, 20]. It is also likely that oral manifestations of other sexually transmitted infections may be concurrently present in those with fellatio-induced mucosal trauma [9, 12, 13, 15, 19–21].

Differential Diagnosis of Fellatio-Associated Oral Lesions

Differential diagnosis of palatal petechiae and purpura includes blood dyscrasia (e.g. disseminated intravascular coagulation, haemophilia, idiopathic thrombocytopenic purpura and leukaemia), infections (e.g. infectious mononucleosis, measles and streptococcal infections), traumatic lesions (e.g. thermal, physical or chemical injuries), medication-induced lesions (e.g. anticoagulant therapy) and neoplasms (e.g. nasopharyngeal carcinoma and Kaposi's sarcoma). If the diagnosis of fellatio-associated mucosal trauma cannot be established, additional evaluation might include complete blood cell counts with platelets and other coagulation studies to examine for blood dyscrasias, serologic studies and cultures for Epstein–Barr virus and β-haemolytic *Streptococcus* infections, and radiographic studies (conventional radiographs, computerised axial tomography and/or magnetic resonance imaging) to examine for neoplasms [19, 22]. All these additional measures are not required on a routine basis.

Clinical Features of Oral Injuries Associated with Cunnilingus

Cunnilingus is also known to cause oral trauma. The lingual frenulum is vulnerable to ulceration by repeated friction during sexual activity (cunnilingus tongue). This is characterised by a horizontal ulceration due to the repetitive scraping of the lingual frenulum against the incisal edges of the mandibular central incisors as the tongue is thrust forward in the sexual act [23]. This lesion usually corresponds to the contact of the ventral tongue with the incisal edge of the mandibular incisor teeth when the tongue is in its most forward position and the lingual frenulum is stretched [23]. The ulceration has a non-specific appearance and is covered with a fibrinous exudate. Ulcer usually resolves in 7–10 days but may recur with repeated performances (Figure 10.2). Over a long period of time, this sexual practice may cause a linear band of fibrous hyperplastic lesion [23].

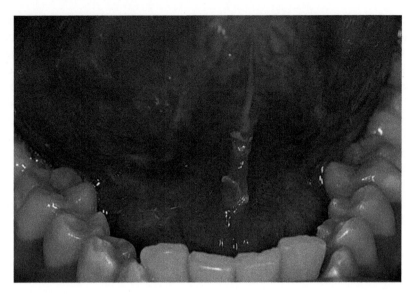

Figure 10.2 Ulceration due to cunnilingus. Ulceration of the lingual frenum caused by repeated trauma from the mandibular incisors as the tongue is thrust forward. Source: Neville et al. [23]. Reproduced with permission from Elsevier.

Differential Diagnosis of Cunnilingus-Associated Oral Lesions

Differential diagnosis includes all forms of traumatic ulcers involving the frenulum. These include traumatic ulcers caused by trauma derived from prosthetic appliances, accidental mechanical injuries, and thermal and chemical injuries. Minor recurrent aphthous ulcers may also be seen on the frenulum in a linear fashion. Differential diagnosis of the cunnilingus-associated fibrous hyperplasia of the lingual frenulum includes keratotic lesions, irritation fibroma and human papillomavirus (HPV)-associated exophytic lesions.

Oral Injuries Associated with Analingus

Analingus can transmit certain sexually transmitted infections to the oral tissues (see Chapter 9), but oral traumatic injuries due to analingus have not been reported.

Diagnosis, Treatment and Prevention of Traumatic Lesions Associated with Oral Sex

A comprehensive history and detailed oral examination are essential to obtain an accurate diagnosis. Usually, treatment of fellatio-induced palatal lesions is not necessary [19–22, 24–26]. Lesions usually heal in a week in the absence of repeated fellatio. Lesions may recur during new episodes of receptive oral sex. Treatment of cunnilingus-associated ulcers of the frenulum may require application of topical anaesthetic cream to relieve symptoms. Fibrous lesions may require surgical excision [23]. The incisal edges of the mandibular teeth can be smoothed to minimise the chance of trauma. Patient education is an important component of the overall management protocol. A major responsibility of the dental care professional is to educate the patient [19, 23].

Oral Trauma Due to Child Sexual Abuse

Most frequent forms of child abuse include physical abuse, neglect and sexual abuse. Lesions and diseases related to those abuses often appear in the craniofacial region in 15% of sexual abuse cases [27].

The dynamics of child sexual abuse differ from those of adult sexual abuse. In particular, children rarely disclose sexual abuse immediately after the event. Moreover, disclosure tends to be a process rather than a single episode and is often initiated following a physical complaint or a change in behaviour [28].

Although the oral cavity is a frequent site of sexual abuse in children, visible oral injuries are rare. [27–30]. Some oral signs of sexual abuse include petechiae, erythema and/or erosions particularly, in the area of the union between the hard and soft palates, caused by forced oral sex. Bite marks can occur inside the mouth caused by the victim's own teeth, produed during sexual abuse.

If the victim of sexual assault reports oral sex, it must be recorded and photographed. The perioral area and the oropharynx should be carefully examined for evidence of trauma. Any signs of petechial presence and/or tears of the frenulum need to be documented. If any oral penetration is suspected the buccal mucosa needs to be swabbed, including the areas under the tongue and around the pillars of the fauces. Swabs should be saved for microscopic examination. Dry sterile swabs should be kept under frozen conditions in order to permit DNA identification later. Patients' privacy must always be ensured [27–30].

Oral healthcare providers are required to report injuries that are due to sexual abuse to child protective services in accordance with local or state legal requirements [30].

References

1 Centre for Disease Control and Prevention (2021). STD Risk and Oral Sex. Available at: https://www.cdc.gov/std/healthcomm/stdfact-stdriskandoralsex.htm

2 Saini, R., Saini, S., and Sharma, S. (2010). Oral sex, oral health and orogenital infections. *J. Glob. Infect.* 2: 57–62. [PMID: 20300419].

3 Habel, M.A., Leichliter, J.S., Dittus, P.J. et al. (2018). Heterosexual anal and Oral sex in adolescents and adults in the United States, 2011–2015. *Sex. Transm. Dis.* 45 (12): 775–782.

4 Conard, L.A. and Blythe, M.J. (2003). Sexual function, sexual abuse and sexually transmitted diseases in adolescence. *Best Pract. Res. Clin. Obstet. Gynaecol.* 17: 103–116. [PubMed] [Google scholar].

5 Remez, L. (2000). Oral sex among adolescents: is it sex or is it abstinence? *Fam. Plann. Perspect.* 32: 298–304. [PubMed] [Google Scholar].

6 Halpern-Felsher, B.L., Cornell, J.L., Kropp, R.Y., and Tschann, J.M. (2005). Oral versus vaginal sex among adolescents: perceptions, attitudes, and behavior. *Pediatrics* 115: 845–851.

7 Boekeloo, B.O. and Howard, D.E. (2002). Oral sexual experience among young adolescents receiving general health examinations. *Am. J. Health Behav.* 26: 306–314. [PubMed] [Google Scholar].

8 Schwartz, I.M. (1999). Sexual activity prior to coital initiation: a comparison between males and females. *Arch. Sex. Behav.* 8: 63–69. [PubMed] [Google scholar].

9 Worsaae, N. and Wanscher, B. (1978). Oral injury caused by fellatio. *Acta Derm. Venereol.* 58: 187–188.

10 Aloi, F.G. (1984). Suffused ecchymosis of the palate caused by fellatio. *G. Ital. Dermatol. Venereol.* 119: 351–352. [PMID: 6510957].

11 Bellizzi, R., Krakow, A.M., and Plack, W. (1980). Soft palate trauma associated with fellatio: case report. *Mil. Med.* 145: 787–788. [PMID: 6783990].

12 van Wyk, C.W. (1981). The oral lesion caused by fellatio. *Am. J. Forensic Med. Pathol.* 2: 217–219. [PMID: 7325131].

13 Muthu, K., Kannan, S., Muthusamy, S., and Sidhu, P. (2015). Palatal ecchymosis associated with irrumation. *Indian J. Dermatol. Venereol. Leprol.* 81 (5): 505–507. https://doi.org/10.4103/0378-6323.162343. PMID: 26261150.

14 Damm, D.D., White, D.K., and Brinker, C.M. (1981). Variations of palatal erythema secondary to fellatio. *Oral Surg. Oral Med. Oral Pathol.* 52: 417–421. [PMID: 6946365] 3.

15 Shanel-Hogan, K.A. (2004). What is this red mark? [signs of abuse]. *J. Calif. Dent. Assoc.* 32: 304–305. [PMID: 15186059].

16 Hupp, W.S. (2009). Palatal erythema. [clinical practice-diagnoistic challenge]. *J. Am. Dent. Assoc.* 140: 555–557. [PMID: 19411524].

17 Farman, A.G. and van Wyk, C.W. (1977). The features of noninfectious oral lesions caused by fellatio. *J. Dent. Assoc. S. Afr.* 1977 (32): 53–55.

18 Heitzler, G.D., Cranin, A.N., and Gallo, L. (1994). Sexual abuse of the oral cavity in children. *N. Y. State Dent.* 60: 31–33. [PMID: 8139820].

19 Cohen, P.R. and Miller, V.M. (2013). Fellatio-associated petechiae of the palate: report of purpuric palatal lesions developing after oral sex. *Dermatol. Online J.* 19 (7): 8.

20 Schlesinger, S.L., Borbotsina, J., and O'Neill, L. (1975). Petechial hemorrhages of the soft palate secondary to fellatio. *Oral Surg. Oral Med. Oral Pathol.* 40: 376–378. [PMID: 1080847].

21 de Barros, L., Grifoni, P., and Navarro, C.M. (2020). Oral lesion secondary to oral sex. Oral surgery, oral medicine, oral pathology and oral Radiology. 129 (1): e67. https://doi.org/10.1016/j.oooo.2019.06.262.

22 Cohen, M.S., Shugars, D.C., and Fiscus, S.A. (2000). Limits on oral transmission of HIV-1. *Lancet* 356: 272. https://doi.org/10.1016/S0140-6736(00)02500-9.

23 Neville, B.W., Damm, D.D., Allen, C.M., and Chi, A.C. (2019). Physical and chemical injuries. In: *Color Atlas of Oral and Maxillofacial Diseases* (ed. B.W. Neville, D.D. Damm, C.M. Allen and A.C. Chi), 169–203. Elsevier.

24 Giansanti, J.S., Cramer, J.R., and Weathers, D.R. (1975). Palatal erythema: another etiologic factor. *Oral Surg. Oral Med. Oral Pathol.* 40: 379–381. [PMID: 1080848].

25 Mendez, L.A., Martinez, R., and Rubio, M. (2018). Fellatio-associated erythema of the soft palate: an incidental finding during a routine dental evaluation. *BMJ Case Rep.* bcr2017221901. https://doi.org/10.1136/bcr-2017-221901.

26 Oliveira, S.C., Slot, D.E., and Van der Weijden, G.A. (2013). What is the cause of palate lesions? A case report. *Int. J. Dent. Hyg.* 11: 306–309.

27 Carlos, A., de la Parte-Sernaa, G., Oliván-Gonzalvob, C.R. et al. (2020). The dark side of Paediatric dentistry: child abuse. *Iberoamerican J. Med.* 03: 194–200.

28 WHO (2021).Child sexual abuse. https://www.who.int/violence_injury_prevention/ resources/publications/en/guidelines_chap7.pdf

29 Costacurta, M., Benavoli, D., Arcudi, G., and Docimo, R. (2016). Oral and dental signs of child abuse and neglect. *Oral Implantol.* 8 (2–3): 68–73. https://doi.org/10.11138/ orl/2015.8.2.068.

30 Fisher-Owens, S.A., Lukefahr, J.L., and Tate, A.R. (2017). Oral and dental aspects of child abuse and neglect. *Pediatr. Dent.* 39 (4): 278–283.

11

Opportunistic Infections, Neoplasms, and Other Oral Lesions in HIV/AIDS

Samuel Sprague, Henry Fan and Newell W. Johnson

Menzies Health Institute Queensland & School of Medicine and Dentistry, Griffith University, Gold Coast, Australia

Introduction

Since the beginning of the HIV epidemic, the importance of oral manifestations has been well documented. Long since established as 'sentinels and signposts' that provide inquisitive clinicians with an early indication of the underlying diseases that human immunodeficiency virus (HIV) and the ensuing immunosuppression inflicts, they also serve as indicators for treatment failure in the era of anti-HIV therapy.

These oral manifestations reflect the degree of immunosuppression in the patient, rather than the mode of acquisition of the virus. Nevertheless, brief consideration of the risk of disease transmission from oral fluids and via the mouth is in order.

The Centres for Disease Control in the USA (https://www.cdc.gov/std/healthcomm/stdfact-stdriskandoralsex.htm) summarises the situation, slightly paraphrased thus: The risk of HIV transmission through oral sex is less of a risk than that of unprotected receptive penile–anal sexual exposure (0.1–3% per episode) or receptive penile–vaginal exposure (0.1–0.2%). Saliva inhibits HIV infectivity and has been shown to kill up to 90% of HIV infected cells and break apart HIV into non-infectious components, so that transmission by kissing or from dental instruments contaminated with saliva is almost unknown. However, if HIV+ [lymphocyte] cells remain present there is a theoretical possibility of transmission from these through the oral mucosa during flossing and/or any other trauma to oral tissues. Several co-factors may increase the risk of HIV transmission as a result of receptive oral sex, including bleeding gums and oral ulcers".

More than 25 HIV associated oral disorders, usually with visible lesions, have been described. Clinically, these oral manifestations of HIV present a twofold challenge for health professionals. Firstly, patients living with HIV more often suffer from stressors – including physical, mental, social and financial challenges – which can lead to neglected dental care, so that these lesions may be discovered with already present dental caries and periodontal problems. Secondly, the clinical course of these common diseases may differ

Sexually Transmissible Oral Diseases, First Edition.
Edited by S.R. Prabhu, Nicholas van Wagoner, Jeff Hill and Shailendra Sawleshwarkar.
© 2023 John Wiley & Sons Ltd. Published 2023 by John Wiley & Sons Ltd.

substantially in those living with HIV compared to patients not infected by HIV, adding extra complexity to both diagnosis and management.

This complexity is compounded by the diversity that exists among those living with HIV. Stark differences exist between, and within, geographical regions regarding access to anti-HIV drugs, most often referred to as antiretroviral therapy (ART), and access to and compliance with ART changes the prevalence of oral manifestations [1].

Health professionals should be suspicious when a new oral lesion is discovered, or an existing condition worsens in an HIV-positive person as it may coincide with an increase in their viral load and/or a fall in CD4$^+$ counts. This often warrants reporting to the patient's HIV physician, as an adjustment to their ART regimen may be required.

When managing oral manifestations of HIV, referral to an oral medicine specialist may be needed and, due to the complexity of drug regimens, treatment should be planned in conjunction with the patient's HIV physician.

It should be noted that it is common for HIV-positive people to be unaware of their HIV status. As with access to ART, regional variation exists with a greater proportion of people unknowingly carrying the infection in developing nations; for example it is estimated that 47% of those living with HIV in Indonesia are unaware [2]. Rates in developed countries, while lesser, are still substantial, such as in the United States with an estimated 15% of individuals who have acquired HIV being unaware of their status [3]. It is prudent for health professionals to keep this in mind when diagnosing oral signs and symptoms that are discussed in this chapter, as they may provide the first clue to a potential HIV diagnosis.

Epidemiology

Early in the HIV epidemic, oral medicine specialists collectively published a document classifying the oral manifestations of HIV and, importantly for clinicians, outlining their diagnostic criteria [4]. Published in 1993, manifestations were sorted based on how common the lesion was seen in people known to be living with HIV (Table 11.1). This classification found wide international acceptance for many years; it is less strictly adhered to now as the epidemic has waned in many countries.

As mentioned previously, the use of ART changes the frequency of oral manifestations and since 1993 considerable shifts in prevalence have been documented. To get a sense of current epidemiological trends, it is prudent to shorten this list to the 10 oral manifestations encountered most frequently (Table 11.2).

Oral candidiasis (OC) has the highest prevalence of any oral manifestation of HIV, and this has remained true since the start of the pandemic. OC is more prevalent among persons with HIV in Africa and Asia (52% and 39%, respectively) than America and Europe (30% and 29%, respectively). Access to ART is known to reduce the occurrence of OC with a lower prevalence among those on ART (26%) than those not on therapy (39%) [5].

Table 11.1 EC Clearinghouse 1993 Classification of Oral Diseases in HIV Infection.

Lesions strongly associated with HIV infection:
- Candidiasis
  - Erythematous
  - Pseudomembranous
- Hairy leukoplakia
- Kaposi's sarcoma
- Non-Hodgkin's lymphoma
- Periodontal disease
  - Linear gingival erythema
  - Necrotising (ulcerative) gingivitis
  - Necrotising (ulcerative) periodontitis

Lesions less commonly associated with HIV infection:
- Bacterial infection
  - *Mycobacterium avium intracellulare*
  - *Mycobacterium tuberculosis*
- Melanotic hyperpigmentation
- Necrotising (ulcerative) stomatitis
- Salivary gland disease
  - Dry mouth due to decreased salivary flow rate
  - Unilateral or bilateral swelling of major salivary glands
- Thrombocytopenic purpura
- Ulceration not otherwise specified (NOS)
- Viral infection
  - Herpes simplex virus
  - Human papillomavirus (warty-like lesions)
    - Condyloma acuminata
    - Focal epithelial hyperplasia
    - Verruca vulgaris
  - Varicella-zoster virus
    - Herpes zoster
    - Varicella

Lesions seen in HIV infection:
- Bacterial infections
  - *Actinomyces israelii*
  - *Escherichia coli*
  - *Klebsiella pneumoniae*
- Cat-scratch disease
- Drug reactions (ulcerative, erythema multiforme, lichenoid and toxic epidermolysis)
- Epithelioid (bacillary) angiomatosis

(Continued)

Table 11.1 (Continued)

- Fungal infection other than candidiasis
  - *Cryptococcus neoformans*
  - *Geotrichum candidum*
  - *Histoplasma capsulatum*
  - *Mucoraceae (mucormycosis/zygomycosis)*
  - *Aspergillus flavus*
- Neurological disturbances
  - Facial palsy
  - Trigeminal neuralgia
- Recurrent aphthous stomatitis
- Viral infections
  - Cytomegalovirus
  - Molluscum contagiosum

Source: William [4]. Republished with permission of John Wiley& Sons.

Table 11.2 Prevalence of oral manifestations of HIV by continent.

Type of oral condition	America (%)	Europe (%)	Africa (%)	Asia (%)
Oral candidiasis	30	29	52	39
Oral hairy leukoplakia	17	16	11	12
Periodontitis and gingivitis	4.4	9.3	8	14
Necrotising ulcerative lesions	2	3	4	2.7
Herpes simplex	3	3	4	10
Aphthous ulcer	5	10	7	9
Non-specific ulceration	4	5	6	7
Kaposi's sarcoma	2	3	14	4
Salivary gland disease	5	10	8	15
Oral warts	2	5	4	0
Oral melanotic hyperpigmentation	8	4	9	21

Source: Tappuni [5] / John Wiley & Sons / CC BY-4.0.

Oral hairy leukoplakia (OHL) is the second most common oral manifestation in most regions. Although ART is known to reduce OHL prevalence considerably [5], it is surprising that studies looking at the prevalence of OHL show higher rates in developed countries than in developing countries (16% and 14%, respectively). This is likely because studies in developed countries are largely done on men who have sex with men (MSM), whereas, in developing countries, the study populations tend to be composed of relatively more heterosexuals, and indeed, more women than men are HIV positive; it is believed that OHL is more common in MSM populations [6, 16].

Of the 10 most common manifestations, 4 show a higher prevalence in patients on ART; these include periodontitis, aphthous ulcers, non-specific ulcers and lesions of herpes simplex [6, 16]. The differences in prevalence are small and causation is difficult to determine. Several contributing factors have been suggested, such as the extended lifespan of many HIV-positive patients with modern care, genetic factors, general oral health, alcohol consumption and diet.

Other notable epidemiological trends include a relatively high prevalence of herpes simplex, salivary gland disease and oral melanotic hyperpigmentation in Asia and a high prevalence of Kaposi's sarcoma (KS) in Africa where the latter remains the most prevalent acquired immune deficiency syndrome (AIDS) defining condition [6, 16].

Oral Opportunistic Infections

HIV-related opportunistic infections are defined as infections that are more frequent or more severe because of immunosuppression mediated by a patient's HIV infection. These include infections with fungal, bacterial and viral aetiologies. Only a subset of these infections presents with oral manifestations but, as noted above, these are common, and effective treatment requirements may be different than in HIV-negative patients.

Fungi

OC is common in patients with HIV infection. *Candida albicans* is the most common species causing infection, although other species such as *Candida glabrata* and *Candida dubliniensis* have been described [6]. *C. albicans* is a dimorphic fungus and exists commensally in the oral cavity.

Four forms of OC have been described in HIV infection: pseudomembranous candidiasis, erythematous candidiasis, angular cheilitis and hyperplastic candidiasis.

Pseudomembranous candidiasis is the most common form of OC in people living with HIV. It presents with lesions that are yellow white, loosely adherent and located anywhere in the mouth (Figure 11.1). Plaques can be wiped away, typically revealing a red mucosa underneath. Clinical diagnosis is usually based on the characteristic appearance of the lesions; however, scrapings can be examined microscopically if further confirmation is needed. Culture is rarely necessary.

Erythematous candidiasis manifests as painful erythematous patches on mucosal surfaces (Figure 11.2) and depapillation on the dorsum of the tongue.

Angular cheilitis presents with erythematous or ulcerated fissures at the commissures of the lips.

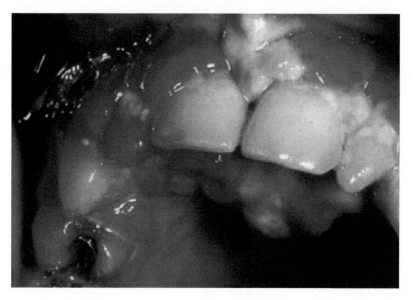

Figure 11.1 Pseudomembranous candidiasis can be seen in this AIDS patient with thrush deposits covering the gingivae and tooth surfaces.

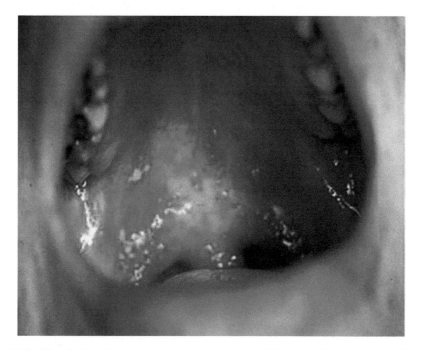

Figure 11.2 Thrush deposits on an erythematous base are visible on the hard and soft palates of this patient, suggesting a diagnosis of erythematous candidiasis.

Hyperplastic candidiasis (previously known as candidal leukoplakia) is the least common form of *Candida* infection in people living with HIV; it typically presents with white patches that are adherent to mucosa.

For OC as it is as effective, more convenient and usually better tolerated than topical therapy [7]. One to two weeks of therapy is recommended. If indicated, various preparations of miconazole, clotrimazole, posaconazole and itraconazole are available and show similar efficacy. Topical preparations are recommended in pregnant patients. Response to treatment typically occurs within 72 hours (for more information see Chapter 18).

Histoplasmosis

It is caused by *Histoplasma capsulatum*, a soil fungus common in the Central and South-central United States, Latin America, the Caribbean and less common in other parts of the world. About half of histoplasmosis cases present with oral lesions [16]. When present, lesions appear as ill-defined ulcerations with a granulomatous surface [8] (Figure 11.3). These can occur anywhere in the mouth. If histoplasmosis is suspected, patients should be sent to an HIV specialist for further diagnosis and therapy, as systemic involvement is possible. Oral lesions can be treated with preparations of ketoconazole and amphotericin B, preferably systemically.

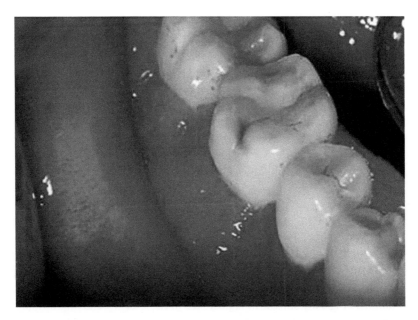

Figure 11.3 An infection by *Histoplasma capsulatum* causing granular inflammation of the free and attached gingiva.

Cryptococcosis

It is usually the result of infection by *Cryptococcus neoformans*; however, *Cryptococcus gattii*, which is found in Australia and similar subtropical regions, can also be a cause. Oral lesions are rare but, if they occur, they appear as ulcerations. Cryptococcosis is severe; diagnosis should be confirmed, and treatment managed by HIV specialists.

Bacteria

Necrotizing Ulcerative Gingivitis (NUG)

It is a condition characterised by destruction of one or more interdental papillae, usually extending to the marginal gingival tissues. It has an acute clinical presentation with interdental gingival necrosis, gingival pain, bleeding, regional lymph node enlargement, fever and halitosis. HIV infection is thought to play a major role in a patient's susceptibility to NUG, although stress and nutritional deficiencies are likely factors as well. *Treponema* spp., *Selenomonas* spp., *Fusobacterium* spp. and *Prevotella intermedia* are found in lesions associated with NUG [9].

Diagnosis can usually be made on clinical signs and symptoms alone. Treatment includes debridement and chemical detersion of necrotic tissue, antiseptic mouth rinses, systemic broad-spectrum antibiotics, analgesics, and scaling and root planing. Concurrent empirical antifungal treatment should be considered to prevent *Candida* super-infection as a result of antibiotic use.

Extension of NUG to bone may cause necrosis; this is termed necrotizing ulcerative periodontitis, and presents with extreme pain and destruction of periodontal attachment – advanced disease will present with exposed bone and even exfoliation of teeth in the involved area. This is rare in developed nations but remains a real problem in less-developed countries, especially in Africa. Specific treatment is the same as for NUG, but patients are likely to be quite febrile, requiring fluid maintenance and analgesics.

Similarly, if NUG progresses to adjacent soft tissues, it is termed necrotizing ulcerative stomatitis (NUS). This presents with acute and painful necrotic lesions of the oral mucosa. Treatment remains the same. Although epidemiological evidence is scant, NUS can progress to Noma (aka cancrum oris), a truly devastating full-thickness necrosis of orofacial soft tissues.

Bacillary Angiomatosis

It is an infection triggered by *Bartonella quintana* – associated with body louse infection and homelessness – and *Bartonella henselae* – associated with exposure to cats. The infection is rare, especially among patients on anti-HIV therapy, but can occur in patients without access to ART, non-compliant to ART or with a late diagnosis of HIV infection. Oral lesions have been described as raised, red–violet, and nodular in appearance. Lesions are clinically and histologically similar in appearance to those of KS, making misdiagnosis a possibility. Erythromycin or doxycycline is considered first-line treatment [10, 11].

Tuberculous (TB) Infection

Tuberculosis is an infection which may occur when a person inhales droplets containing *Mycobacterium tuberculosis*. In the modern age, tuberculosis is curable, and great efforts have been made to prevent spread but, despite these efforts, tuberculosis remains the leading cause of morbidity and mortality among those living with HIV [12]. After acquisition and primary infection, tuberculosis typically remains in a latent stage until a patient is immunosuppressed; at that point, they may develop systemic disease. Oral lesions during primary infection are rare and more common in children; they appear as a single painless ulcer. In secondary infection, lesions are more common and may present as single or multiple ulcers with irregular borders, minimal induration and an irregular periphery (Figure 11.4). Classical 'cold abscess', with fistula, may develop from draining lymph nodes in the submandibular or cervical chain.

As signs and symptoms of TB are largely non-specific and suggestive of systemic disease, and open oral or skin lesions are contagious, any suspicion of tubercular infection should result in immediate referral to an infectious disease physician. Treatment is typically initiated based on a clinical diagnosis, but a confirmatory culture will also be done. Current treatment includes a four-drug regimen of isoniazid, rifampin, ethambutol and pyrazinamide [12].

Mycobacterium avium Complex (MAC) Infection

This infection is thought to be acquired through inhalation, ingestion or inoculation of bacteria of the MAC via the respiratory or gastrointestinal tract. The disease occurs in the most immunosuppressed patients and typically presents as a disseminated infection. Oral lesions are very rare but when present they can be seen as a granulomatous mass.

Viruses

Human Herpesviruses

Herpes simplex virus (*HSV*) infection, which encompasses infections caused by human HSV type 1 (HSV-1) and type 2 (HSV-2), both of which are alphaherpesvirinae, is common with

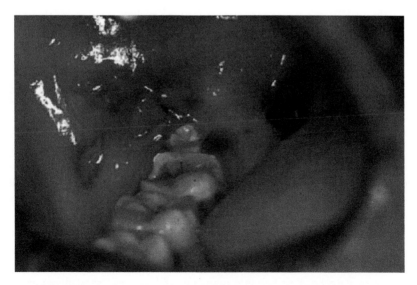

Figure 11.4   Identifiable in the retromolar area of this person with AIDS are punched-out ulcers due to tuberculosis infection. This patient had disseminated tuberculosis with multiple visceral lesions and 'cold abscesses' draining from infected lymph nodes.

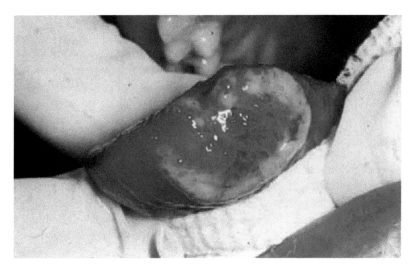

Figure 11.5 Herpes simplex virus infection causing severe ulceration of the tongue in this HIV-positive patient.

an estimated two-thirds of the world population infected with HSV-1 and 13% infected with HSV-2 [13]. One form of HSV infection is primary herpetic gingivostomatitis, which may be seen in susceptible children or adolescents, but this is uncommon in HIV-infected adults. On the other hand, recurrent oral herpes, another manifestation of HSV infection, is common among those living with HIV.

In patients with HIV, recurrent herpetic infection presents with painful, large ulcers (Figure 11.5). These can be found anywhere in the oral cavity and, unlike the ulcers in patients without HIV, the ulcers may persist for long periods – failure of these ulcers to resolve in four weeks is considered AIDS defining.

Diagnosis can be based on clinical findings; however, if in doubt, a laboratory diagnosis should be pursued. Polymerase chain reaction of HSV deoxyribonucleic acid (DNA) and viral culture are the preferred methods for confirmatory diagnosis. Treatment of episodes can include systemic acyclovir, valacyclovir or famciclovir. Topical preparations are not effective for oral lesions.

Herpes zoster, also known as shingles, is caused by reactivation of the varicella-zoster virus (VZV: another alphaherpesvirus, also known as HHV-3) – the infecting agent in chickenpox. Herpes zoster occurs in the general population, especially among the elderly; however, those living with HIV have a more than fourfold greater risk of developing this condition [14]. The rash associated with herpes zoster follows a dermatomal distribution and evolves in stages of macules, papules, vesicles, pustules and crusts.

Oral lesions are typically unilateral and painful. They appear as erosive spots that coalesce to form ulcers. The facial skin along a dermatome of the trigeminal nerve may be affected (Figure 11.6). In cases of trigeminal nerve involvement, the patient may complain of toothache or earache. Post-herpetic neuralgia and systemic viral dissemination are feared complications. Preferred treatment options include valacyclovir and famciclovir for 7 10 days – longer durations may be required if lesions heal slowly.

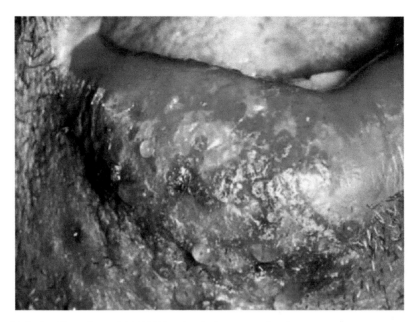

Figure 11.6 In this patient with HIV blistering lesions caused by herpes zoster virus can be seen. Lesions were present across the skin of the lower face, implicating the mandibular branch of the trigeminal nerve.

Epstein–Barr virus (EBV), a gammaherpesvirus, also known as HHV-4, is an exceedingly common virus worldwide with some estimates suggesting a lifetime prevalence of 90% [15]. The initial infection is often subclinical but commonly presents as infectious mononucleosis (glandular fever).

In an oral context, especially among those living with HIV, EBV is the cause of OHL. While possible in immunosuppression generally, OHL is a renowned early marker of HIV infection. Often asymptomatic, it presents as a unilateral or bilateral non-painful white lesion, which is most often present on the lateral border of the tongue (Figures 11.7 and 11.8). Its range of appearance includes a smooth, flat, and small lesion – typically when present on areas other than the lateral tongue – to a 'hairy' irregular lesion with folds and projections. Unlike the most common presentation of OC, it is an adherent lesion that cannot be removed by scraping.

If a patient is known to be HIV positive, a diagnosis of OHL can be made based on the clinical appearance. EBV can also be tested for in epithelial cells, usually by in situ hybridisation techniques, if definitive diagnosis is required. Due to the benign nature of OHL, treatment is generally not required. Regardless, if treatment is desired – as may be requested by the patient for aesthetic reasons ART is the first line of treatment. OHL has been found to respond to oral acyclovir, valacyclovir and famciclovir; however, reoccurrence after the cessation of treatment is common. Topical treatment with podophyllin resin and retinoic acid may be effective, though difficult in the wet environment of the mouth. Lesions may be ablated by cryotherapy, but problems with reoccurance remain.

EBV is also known to drive malignant transformation of epithelial cells and of lymphocytes, as discussed in the following section.

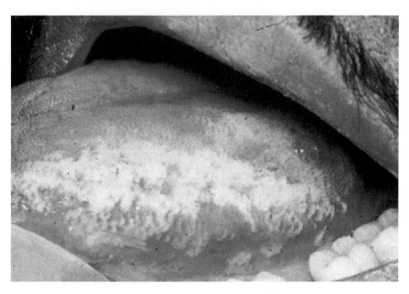

Figure 11.7   The classic presentation of oral hairy leukoplakia with a sizeable white lesion covering the lateral border of the patient's tongue.

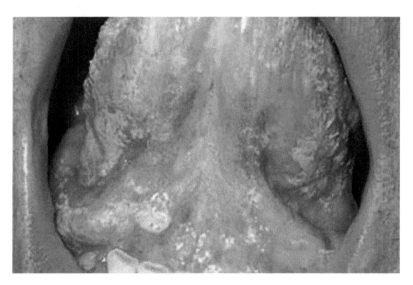

Figure 11.8   Oral hairy leukoplakia presenting white patches on the lateral border of the tongue, the ventral tongue and floor of the mouth mucosa.

Cytomegalovirus (CMV), a betaherpesvirus, also known as human herpesvirus 5 [HHV5], can cause severe disease in people living with HIV, who have advanced immunosuppression. Most often this occurs as a result of a latent infection being reactivated. If oral lesions are present, they are typically innocuous looking but painful ulcers that have a white halo around the necrotic core (Figure 11.9).

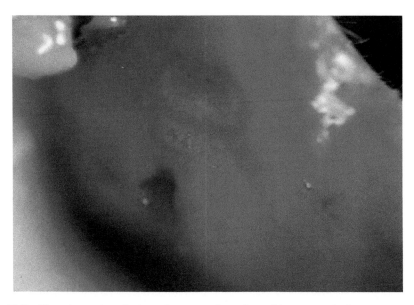

Figure 11.9 Ulcers located on the buccal mucosa of a patient with cytomegalovirus are non-specific in appearance. The deep ulcer could be confused with a tubercular lesion as described above.

Oral ulcers caused by CMV can be easily confused with other ulcerative conditions and, as a rule, if a HIV-positive patient presents with ulcers that do not resolve rapidly, a swab in viral transport medium should be sent to a diagnostic microbiology laboratory for virus identification. If systemic involvement is suspected, they should be sent to a specialist physician for further work-up. If allowed to progress, CMV infection in immunosuppressed patients may cause retinitis, and possibly encephalitis. CMV infection responds to systemic valganciclovir and intravenous ganciclovir, which are considered first-line treatment.

Human herpesvirus 8, another gammaherpesvirus, is the cause of KS, and is presented in the following section of this chapter.

Human Papillomaviruses (HPV)
HPV infections can be the result of infection with any of the over 100 known genotypes of HPV. Certain strains of HPV (particularly HPV-16 and HPV-18) are especially problematic as they act as a driver of several malignancies, including of the oropharynx, and these malignancies are found more often in those living with HIV.

In terms of non-malignancies, two HPV-associated lesions are known to occur in the oral cavity of people with HIV: oral warts and focal epithelial hyperplasia.

Oral warts often referred to as condyloma acuminatum are small asymptomatic lesions that appear as pink or white elevated papules; they are often described as having a flat (Figure 11.10) or cauliflower-like appearance. Focal epithelial hyperplasia presents as a smooth flat-topped lesion with a cobblestone appearance. Both lesions typically present with multiple occurrences, and the associated virus is usually HPV types 13 and/or 32, which cause Heck's disease, relatively common in some HIV-negative populations, such as indigenous populations of North, Central and South America.

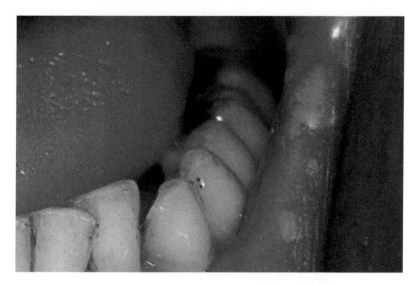

Figure 11.10 Flat condylomata due to HPV infection, located on the vermillion lip mucosa of an HIV-positive patient.

Diagnosis is typically made by visual inspection and only confirmed with biopsy if the diagnosis is uncertain. Surgical, laser and cryotherapy may be used as treatment (For more information see Chapter 15).

Neoplasms

Non-Hodgkin's lymphoma (NHL) and KS are the two major AIDS-defining cancers discussed here in detail. Other non-AIDS-defining cancers include non-small cell lung cancer, Hodgkin's lymphoma, oropharyngeal cancer, hepatocellular carcinoma and squamous cell carcinoma of the anus, vulva and penis [16].

Non-Hodgkin's Lymphomas

NHLs are a group of lymphoproliferative neoplasms. They are more likely to distribute to extranodal tissues compared to Hodgkin's lymphoma. The most prevalent types of NHLs are diffuse large B-cell lymphoma (DLBL) and follicular lymphoma (FL), and over 90% of AIDS-associated NHLs are of B-lymphocyte origin [17].

Australia has the second highest age-standardised incidence rates (ASIR) of NHLs in the world for both men (15.3/100 000) and women (12.3/100 000), but the ASIR has stabilised since the 1990s. The male-to-female ratio varies from 1.1 to 1.8 depending on geographic location [18]. Patients with AIDS are at 100–200 times higher risk of developing NHLs than the general population, and it is estimated that NHLs are found in 5–10% of HIV-infected patients despite decreasing global ASIR after the introduction of combined antiretroviral therapy (cART) [18, 19].

The pathogenesis of NHLs is a multifactorial process generally involving suppressed T-cell function, and latent EBV infection generating prolonged antigen stimulation [17]. HIV/AIDS are well-established risk factors for NHLs, which allow EBV-infected B cells to undergo transformation and excessive proliferation with limited regulation from the immune system [20]. Other risk factors include immunocompromising conditions such as in organ transplant patients, autoimmune disorders and chronic inflammatory diseases [17].

EBV is an icosahedral γ-DNA virus commonly transmitted by oral and respiratory secretions and lies dormant until psychological stress, immunosuppression, including HIV/AIDS allow the virus to reactivate, proliferate and enter a lytic phase [20]. Clinically, NHLs in HIV patients often manifest initially as asymptomatic cervical lymphadenopathy, often with abdominal involvement, while extranodal NHLs, of which the majority of cases are found in Waldeyer's ring, present variously depending on the location of lesions in the head and neck [17]. Signs and symptoms include pain, swelling, tooth displacement, paraesthesia, dysphagia, asymptomatic tonsil enlargement, nasal obstruction and hearing loss [19]. Oral NHLs are seen in advanced HIV/AIDS patients, in which the tumour, often with mucosal ulceration, can be rapidly progressive [17, 19] (Figure 11.11). Differential diagnosis (DDx) of the subtypes of NHLs – small B-cell lymphocytic lymphoma, chronic lymphocytic leukaemia, follicular lymphoma, mantle–cell lymphoma, DLBL and Burkitt's lymphoma, T-cell lymphomas, and precursor B-cell and T-cell lymphomas – requires expert histopathological diagnosis [21].

Different types of NHLs require specific treatments: cyclophosphamide, vincristine, doxorubicin, and prednisolone with/without rituximab are currently used as first-line chemotherapy for DLBL, while FL can be treated by chemotherapy, radiotherapy and haemopoietic stem-cell transplantation [21]. New monoclonal antibody treatments for NHLs have shown positive

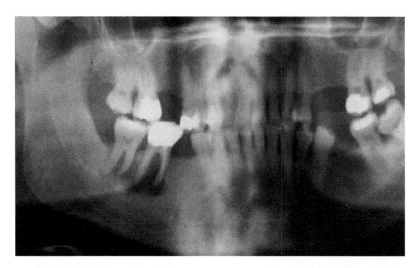

Figure 11.11 The periapical radiolucency associated with the lower right second permanent molar was regarded as infective/inflammatory in origin and the tooth treated by his dental practitioner by root filling and a crown. The lesion did not resolve and biopsy in our oral medicine clinic revealed a NHL. Other lymphomata were identified by whole body imaging.

outcomes, but more evidence is needed. About 30–40% of patients with DLBL will relapse after chemotherapy, and the prognosis depends on initial response to treatment and localization of the cancer [21]. Similarly, histological transformation of FL to diffuse aggressive lymphoma with associated staging determines prognosis. Complications of NHLs include widespread metastasis and obstruction of important vessels [21]. Early diagnosis remains important for good outcomes for patients who develop NHLs as part of their HIV disease.

Kaposi's Sarcoma

KS is an angioproliferative neoplasm caused by productive infection with HHV-8, typically in patients with HIV/AIDS [22]. HHV-8 infection alone, however, is insufficient for the development of KS: genetic, environmental and immunological factors play a part [23]. KS, as an oral manifestation of HIV, has a higher prevalence in Africa (14%) compared to North America (2%), Europe (3%) and Asia (4%), and is frequently observed among MSM [5]. Patients with AIDS are between 300 and 20000 times more likely to develop KS compared to patients solely immunocompromised and the general population, respectively [24]. Geographical variation of the incidence of KS is related to the underlying prevalence of HHV-8 in the community [25]. The ASIR of KS in Australia is less than 0.3/100000, and the seroprevalence rate of HHV-8 is about 6–10%, which is consistent with other developed countries [24]. Africa has a community HHV-8 seroprevalence of 30–80% and the highest ASIR of KS in the world both before and throughout the HIV epidemic [25].

There are four KS variants: classic, endemic, iatrogenic and epidemic (AIDS related). All are causally associated with HHV-8 [23]. Other associated factors described include local and systemic immunodeficiency (notably HIV/AIDS), persistent HHV-8 carriage, and use of anti-malarial medications (e.g. quinine or 4-aminoquinolines), immunomodulators (e.g. chloroquine and hydroxychloroquine) and vasoactive agents (e.g. angiotensin-converting enzyme inhibitors) [23].

HHV-8 possesses the ability to infect epithelial and endothelial cells, monocytes, fibroblasts and perhaps other less well-defined cell types [24]. As a linear DNA gamma herpesvirus with an icosahedral capsid, the viral genome incorporates into host DNA and enters either viral latency or viral lytic replication. Once the virus is activated, it can encode proteins and micro-RNAs that are responsible for oncogenic, anti-apoptotic, immune-modulatory, proinflammatory and angiogenic processes for the development of KS [24]. HIV can activate latent HHV-8, increase its viral load and promote the development of KS. HIV-1 can release a wide range of regulatory proteins, including proangiogenic chemokines, which enhance the growth of HHV-8-infected cells [22, 24]. In the upper aerodigestive tract, HHV-8 reservoirs are the lymphoid mucosae of Waldeyer's ring, so the virus is readily detected in whole mouth fluid [24]. Nevertheless, studies are unable to establish a clear dominant route of viral transmission or factors which influence the incubation period for KS.

Clinical features of KS range from mild skin lesions to extensive visceral involvement, but generally appear as multiple, pink to purple, raised or flat lesions that are usually asymptomatic (Figure 11.12). The lesions can become exophytic and ulcerated [24, 26] (Figure 11.13). Intraoral palatal and gingival lesions are common among patients with uncontrolled AIDS and may lead to dysphagia and secondary infection [24]. Pulmonary, gastrointestinal and other systemic KS lesions can result in severe complications including dyspnoea, haemoptysis, lymphatic obstruction and function-limiting oedema [24, 26].

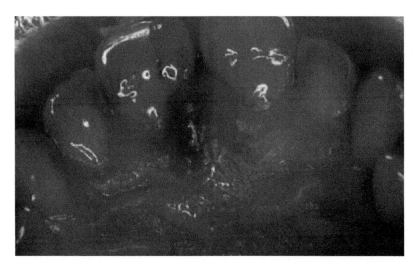

Figure 11.12 A small Kaposi's sarcoma – likely early in its development – can be visualised on the palatal gingiva of this patient.

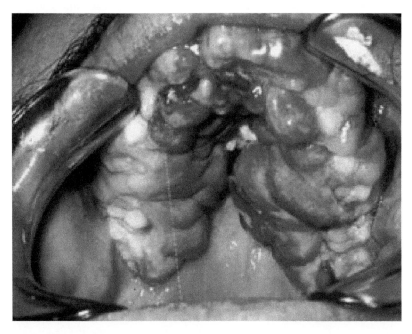

Figure 11.13 An AIDS patient with a massive Kaposi's sarcoma that has encompassed the maxillary gingival tissues.

DDx of KS as a cutaneous lesion are interstitial granuloma annulare, spindle cell hae-mangioma, kaposiform haemangioendothelioma, cutaneous angiosarcoma and aneurys-mal dermatofibroma, while DDx of mucocutaneous lesions are pyogenic granuloma, bacillary angiomatosis, haemangioma and angiosarcoma [26]. All clinically suspicious for KS should have the diagnosis confirmed histologically. Typical features in haematoxylin and eosin (H&E)-stained sections are spindle cell and small vascular proliferations, with extravasated blood and inflammatory cells [27]. Staining for HHV-8 by immunocytochemistry is conclusive [28].

Immune reconstitution of HIV/AIDS with cART is the main treatment for KS, while evidence of the efficacy of other available treatments such as interferon-alpha and alitretinoin remains limited [23, 24, 26]. The five-year survival rate of localised KS is 81%, 62% in regional and 41% in dispersed disease [29]. Early diagnosis allows prompt initiation of cART and improves the prognosis of KS.

Other Lesions

Recurrent aphthous ulcers are generally seen in HIV patients with a previous history of recurrent aphthous stomatitis. Patients will often report an increase in the frequency and severity of episodes.

Caution is advised when determining aetiology for oral ulcerations. Infectious agents must be seriously considered because leaving infections – particularly CMV and other HHVs – untreated in HIV-positive patients may cause severe disease and death.

In cases of recurrent aphthous stomatitis, the minor type is more common in those living with HIV (Figure 11.14), but the major type still occurs. The approach to diagnosis is the same as one would employ in patients without HIV, such as screening for food allergies, particularly gluten sensitivity, haematological abnormalities and inflammatory bowel disease. Similarly, treatments remain the same, with topical steroids and thalidomide as options.

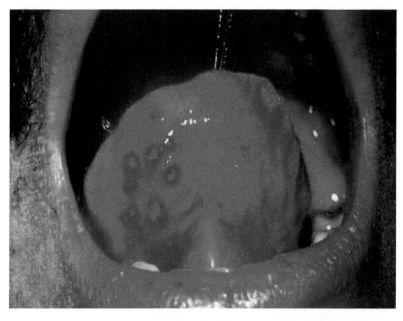

Figure 11.14 An HIV-positive patient with minor aphthous ulcers presenting on the ventral surface of the tongue.

Periodontal disease related to HIV is largely dependent on a patient's immune status, and thus their access to optimal ART and general oral hygiene. As discussed in the '*Oral Opportunistic Infections*' section of this chapter, incidence of necrotizing ulcerative gingivitis, periodontitis, and necrotising stomatitis decreases with adequate anti-HIV therapy.

Linear gingival erythema is a periodontal condition characterised by a red marginal gingivitis of the upper and lower anterior gingivae (Figure 11.15). Its aetiology is debated but it is thought to be a manifestation of candidal growth and is more common in HIV patients with poor oral hygiene.

Salivary gland disease in the context of HIV infection is more common in children than adults [30]. It presents with unilateral or bilateral soft enlargement of the parotid glands and in some cases is painful. There is often associated xerostomia and fever. In patients with known HIV infection, clinical presentation and ultrasound scans are sufficient for diagnosis. The pathogenesis involves T-cell infiltration of the parenchyma. It may be part of wider diffuse infiltrative lymphocytosis syndrome (DILS). Differential diagnosis again involves elimination of infectious agents and neoplasms.

Hyperpigmentation of the oral mucosa is a common finding in longstanding HIV infection [31] (Figure 11.16). This may be drug induced, or Addisonian, following adrenal damage by HIV-associated lymphocyte infiltration. Referral to an endocrinologist is advisable to rule out the possibility of the latter.

In intra-mucosal haemorrhages/purpure, HIV infection often causes marked thrombocytopaenia, particularly in acute or initial phases [32]. This can present as intra-mucosal and conjunctival haemorrhages.

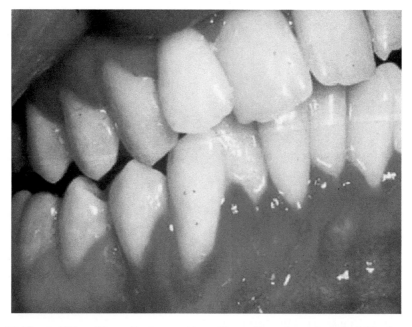

Figure 11.15 An HIV-positive patient presenting with a pattern of marginal gingivitis often classified as linear gingival erythema.

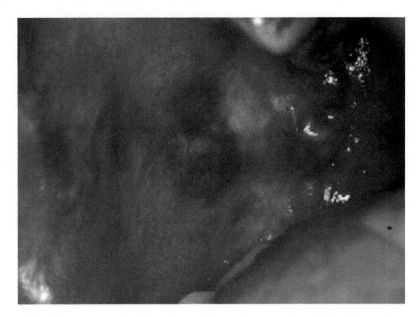

Figure 11.16 Pigmented patches located on the buccal mucosa in an HIV-positive patient.

Immune Reconstitution Inflammatory Syndrome (IRIS)

In IRIS, a recovering immune system responds to an extant infection by raising cell-mediated inflammation [33]. This may happen when an AIDS patient begins Active Antiretroviral Therapy (ART). Concurrent treatment of the infection is important. Infections commonly associated with IRIS include cytomegalovirus, herpes zoster, MAC, Pneumocystis pneumonia, and *M. tuberculosis*. Associated oral infections include HHV-8, *Candida* and HPV with oral warts.

Acknowledgements

Authors wish to thank John Wiley & Sons and the Editor of Australian Dental Journal for granting us permission to reproduce images from: Johnson, N.W. (2010). *The Mouth in HIV/AIDS: Marker of Disease Status and Management Challenges for the Dental Profession.* Aust. Dental J. *55*(Suppl 1(s1)):85–102.

References

1 Khoury, Z.H. and Meeks, V. (2021). The influence of antiretroviral therapy on HIV-related oral manifestations. *J. Natl. Med. Assoc.* 113 (4): 449–456.
2 Riono, P. and Challacombe, S.J. (2020). HIV in Indonesia and in neighbouring countries and its social impact. *Oral Dis.* 26 (S1): 28–33.

3 Satcher Johnson, A., Song, R., and Hall, H.I. (2017). Estimated HIV incidence, prevalence, and undiagnosed infections in US states and Washington, DC, 2010–2014. *JAIDS J. Acquired Immune Deficiency Syndr.* 76 (2): 116–122.

4 (1993). Williams D. M. Classification and diagnostic criteria for oral lesions in HIV infection. EC-clearinghouse on oral problems related to HIV infection and WHO collaborating Centre on oral manifestations of the immunodeficiency virus. *J. Oral Pathol. Med.* 22 (7): 289–291.

5 Tappuni, A.R. (2020). The global changing pattern of the oral manifestations of HIV. *Oral Dis.* 26 (S1): 22–27.

6 Johnson, N.W. (2010). The mouth in HIV/AIDS: markers of disease status and management challenges for the dental profession. *Aust. Dent. J.* 55: 85–102.

7 Rajadurai, S.G., Maharajan, M.K., Veettil, S.K., and Gopinath, D. (2021). Comparative efficacy of antifungal agents used in the treatment of oropharyngeal candidiasis among HIV-infected adults: a systematic review and network meta-analysis. *J. Fungi* 7 (8): 637.

8 Ferreira, O.G., Cardoso, S.V., Borges, A.S. et al. (2002). Oral histoplasmosis in Brazil. *Oral Surg. Oral Med. Oral Pathol. Oral Radiol. Endod.* 93 (6): 654–659.

9 Malek, R., Gharibi, A., Khlil, N., and Kissa, J. (2017). Necrotizing ulcerative gingivitis. Contemporary. *Clin. Dent.* 8 (3): 496.

10 Koehler, J.E., Sanchez, M.A., Garrido, C.S. et al. (1997). Molecular epidemiology of bartonella infections in patients with bacillary angiomatosis–peliosis. *N. Engl. J. Med.* 337 (26): 1876–1883.

11 Blanc, S.L., Sambuelli, R., Femopase, F. et al. (2000). Bacillary angiomatosis affecting the oral cavity. Report of two cases and review. *J. Oral Pathol. Med.* 29 (2): 91–96.

12 Kant, S., Sharma, S., Bajpai, J. et al. (2019). Oral tuberculosis – current concepts. *J. Family Med. Primary Care* 8 (4): 1308.

13 James, C., Harfouche, M., Welton, N.J. et al. (2020). Herpes simplex virus: global infection prevalence and incidence estimates, 2016. *Bull. World Health Organ.* 98 (5): 315–329.

14 Jansen, K., Haastert, B., Michalik, C. et al. (2013). Incidence and risk factors of herpes zoster among HIV-positive patients in the German Competence Network for HIV/AIDS (KompNet): a cohort study analysis. *BMC Infect. Dis.* 13 (1): 372. https://doi.org/10.1186/1471-2334-13-372.

15 Fugl, A. and Andersen, C.L. (2019). Epstein–Barr virus and its association with disease – a review of relevance to general practice. *BMC Fam. Pract.* 20 (1): 62.

16 Johnson, N.W., Anaya-Saavedra, G., and Webster-Cyriaque, J. (2020). Viruses and oral diseases in HIV-infected individuals on long-term antiretroviral therapy: what are the risks and what are the mechanisms? *Oral Dis.* 26 (1): 80–90.

17 Singh, R., Shaik, S., Negi, B.S. et al. (2020). Non-Hodgkin's lymphoma: a review. *J. Family Med. Prim. Care* 9 (4): 1834–1840.

18 Miranda-Filho, A., Piñeros, M., Znaor, A. et al. (2019). Global patterns and trends in the incidence of non-Hodgkin lymphoma. *Cancer Causes Control* 30 (5): 489–499.

19 Silva, T.D.B., Ferreira, C.B.T., Leite, G.B. et al. (2016). Oral manifestations of lymphoma: a systematic review. *Ecancermedicalscience* 10: 665.

20 Kerr, J.R. (2019). Epstein–Barr virus (EBV) reactivation and therapeutic inhibitors. *J. Clin. Pathol.* 72 (10): 651–658.

21 Shankland, K.R.D., Armitage, J.O.P., and Hancock, B.W.P. (2012). Non-Hodgkin lymphoma. *The Lancet (British Edition)* 380 (9844): 848–857.

22 Curtiss, P., Strazzulla, L.C., and Friedman-Kien, A.E. (2016). An update on Kaposi's sarcoma: epidemiology, pathogenesis and treatment. *Dermatol. Therapy* 6 (4): 465–470.

23 Ruocco, E.M.D.P., Ruocco, V.M.D., Tornesello, M.L.P. et al. (2013). Kaposi's sarcoma: etiology and pathogenesis, inducing factors, causal associations, and treatments: facts and controversies. *Clin. Dermatol.* 31 (4): 413–422.

24 Cesarman, E., Damania, B., Krown, S.E. et al. (2019). Kaposi sarcoma. *Nat. Rev. Dis. Primers.* 5 (1): 9.

25 Dollard, S.C., Butler, L.M., Jones, A.M. et al. (2010). Substantial regional differences in human herpesvirus 8 seroprevalence in sub-Saharan Africa: insights on the origin of the "Kaposi's sarcoma belt". *Int. J. Cancer* 127 (10): 2395–2401.

26 Radu, O. and Pantanowitz, L. (2013). Kaposi sarcoma. *Arch. Pathol. Lab. Med.* 137 (2): 289–294.

27 Fatahzadeh, M. (2012). Kaposi sarcoma: review and medical management update. *Oral Surg. Oral Med. Oral Pathol. Oral Radiol. Endod.* 113 (1): 2–16.

28 Douglas, J.L., Gustin, J.K., Moses, A.V. et al. (2010). Kaposi sarcoma pathogenesis: a triad of viral infection, oncogenesis and chronic inflammation. *Transl. Biomed.* 1 (2): 172.

29 Howlader, N., Noone, A.M., Krapcho, M. (eds). (2020). SEER Cancer Statistics Review, 1975-2017, National Cancer Institute. Bethesda, MD, https://seer.cancer.gov/csr/1975_2017, based on November 2019 SEER data submission, posted to the SEER web site.

30 Frezzini, C., Leao, J.C., and Porter, S. (2005). Current trends of HIV disease of the mouth. *J. Oral Pathol. Med.* 34 (9): 513–531.

31 Feller, L., Chandran, R., Kramer, B. et al. (2014). Melanocyte biology and function with reference to oral melanin hyperpigmentation in HIV-seropositive subjects. *AIDS Res. Hum. Retroviruses* 30 (9): 837–843. http://dx.doi.org/10.1089/aid.2014.0062.

32 Alshamam, M.S., Sumbly, V., Khan, S. et al. (2021). Acquired thrombotic thrombocytopenic purpura in a newly diagnosed HIV patient: a case report and literature review. *Cureus* 13 (6): e15967. https://doi.org/10.7759/cureus.15967.

33 Murdoch, D.M., Venter, W.D., Van Rie, A. et al. (2007). Immune reconstitution inflammatory syndrome (IRIS): review of common infectious manifestations and treatment options. *AIDS Res. Ther.* 4: 9. https://doi.org/10.1186/1742-6405-4-9.

12

Oral Manifestations of Syphilis

Andrea B. Moleri[1], Mário J. Romañach[2], Ana L.O.C. Roza[3] and S.R. Prabhu[4]

[1]Oral Medicine, School of Dentistry, Universidade Federal Fluminense, Niterói, Brazil
[2]Department of Oral Diagnosis and Pathology, School of Dentistry, Universidade Federal do Rio de Janeiro, Rio de Janeiro, Brazil
[3]Department of Oral Diagnosis, Piracicaba Dental School, Universidade Estadual de Campinas, Piracicaba, Brazil
[4]University of Queensland, School of Dentistry, Brisbane, Australia

Introduction

Syphilis is predominantly a sexually transmitted bacterial infection caused by *Treponema pallidum*. It affects many systems of the body including the mouth. Clinical manifestations of sexually acquired syphilis are divided into primary, secondary, and tertiary syphilis. Congenital syphilis (CS) can occur when a mother with syphilis passes the infection on to her baby during pregnancy. Syphilis has been nicknamed as the 'the great imitator' because it mimics a variety of infectious, neoplastic or immune-mediated disorders [1]. Clinical manifestations of syphilis including those of the oral structures often create a diagnostic challenge to the clinician leading to delay in diagnosis or misdiagnosis. Oral manifestations of syphilis may be one of the first signs of the systemic disease. Correct and early diagnosis of oral manifestations is of great importance for the treatment of syphilis [2]. This chapter deals with key features of syphilis, its oral manifestations, diagnosis and management.

Epidemiology

According to the World Health Organization (WHO), approximately 17.7 million individuals aged 15–49 years worldwide had syphilis in 2012, with the highest prevalence observed in Africa [3]. In recent years, the incidence of syphilis has been increasing in the United States and Europe, mainly due to changes in sexual behaviour and decreasing use of barrier protection (i.e. condoms) [4]. In low- and middle-income countries, heterosexual transmission of syphilis remains problematic in some high-risk subpopulations, such as female sex

Sexually Transmissible Oral Diseases, First Edition.
Edited by S.R. Prabhu, Nicholas van Wagoner, Jeff Hill and Shailendra Sawleshwarkar.
© 2023 John Wiley & Sons Ltd. Published 2023 by John Wiley & Sons Ltd.

workers and their male clients [3]. In high-income countries, there was a decrease in the prevalence of syphilis among heterosexuals. However, the disease is more common among men who have sex with men (MSM) [3, 5].

In active syphilis, the primary lesion of syphilis is known as syphilitic chancre. It occurs at the site of inoculation of *T. pallidum* and is more common in the genital region. The most frequent location of extragenital chancre is anal or oral mucosa, with the reported incidence being 5–14% [6]. About two-thirds occur in or around the mouth after unprotected oral sex. Among MSM, 12.5% of syphilitic chancres are oral [7]. Oral sex in recent years has been erroneously considered a safer sexual practice, which does not require the use of protective barriers. This misconception has resulted in an increase in oral lesions of sexually transmitted infections (STIs) including syphilis [7]. Although oral manifestations of syphilis may be observed at all stages of the disease, they are more commonly detected at the secondary stage.

Risk Factors/Predisposing Factors

The increased incidence of STI reflects, in part, the changes in people's behaviour in relation to sexual conduct. Sexual conduct involves different types of experiences and practices. In this context, oral sex has become increasingly popular, which contributes to a corresponding increase in oral and oropharyngeal manifestations of STIs. Oral sex practices such as fellatio, cunnilingus and anilingus allow the transmission of infectious agents from genital and anal regions to the oral cavity and vice versa [1, 7–9].

The practice of oral sex is common in hetero- and same sex relationships. It can cause infectious and traumatic lesions. When the oral mucosa is traumatised, sexually transmissible infectious agents can enter the oral mucosa [7, 9, 10]. The practice of orogenital sex between MSM men and women is almost universal. Data regarding opposite-sex sexual behaviour from a survey show that between 2011 and 2013, in the United States, 86.2% of women and 87.4% of men had oral sex [11]. Syphilis infection has also been associated with several other risk and predisposing factors, which often overlap, such as people who have sex under the influence of psychotropic substances and alcohol, early initiation of sexual activity without educational guidance, poor access to health services, social marginalisation or low socioeconomic and cultural level, and persons deprived of liberty. Syphilis may also occur as a co-infection in HIV-seropositive patients.

Microbiology/Transmission

T. pallidum, the causative bacteria of syphilis is a spiral microorganism unique to the human species. It measures approximately 6–15 μm long and 0.25 μm thick, dimensions below the resolution of brightfield microscopy. The motility and ability of the organism to adhere to cells contribute to its virulence. It is able to pass through intact mucous membrane or abraded skin. The bacteria are sensitive to heat, dry environments, common detergents and antiseptics. *T. Pallidum* does not grow in cultures [1–5].

Syphilis is transmitted by direct contact with an infectious lesion, almost always sexual, or by transplacental passage during pregnancy. In heterosexual patients, bacterial entry is typically genital or oral, but in MSM, transmission of bacteria may often be extragenital (anal, rectal and/or oral). *T. pallidum* does not invade intact skin; however, it can invade intact or abraded mucosal epithelium. To establish infection, *T. pallidum* must adhere to epithelial cells and extracellular matrix components and invade tissues using their motility across intercellular junctions, the so-called 'interjunctional' penetration [3]. In the oral cavity, mucosal abrasions created by oral sex, kissing (bite injuries), sharp edges of dental prosthesis or fractured teeth may facilitate the transmission of syphilis from the infected partner to the uninfected partner. *T. Pallidum* initially multiplies locally and then spreads through the lymphatic and blood stream [4].

Clinical Manifestations

Infected individuals follow a disease course divided into primary, secondary, latent (early and late) and tertiary stages. The guidelines from the United States and Europe define 'early syphilis' as an infection of <1 year in duration, whereas the WHO defines it as an infection <2 years' duration [10]. The WHO has based this division on the infectiousness of syphilis and its response to therapy. Early stages are more infectious but respond better to treatment. In the initial stages, the symptoms are variable and disappear even without treatment.

The incubation period is from 21 to 30 days after the penetration of *T. pallidum*. This can vary from 10 to 90 days, which will depend on the number and virulence of the infecting bacteria and the individual's immune response [2]. Primary syphilis is characterised by the appearance of a chancre [5, 10, 12] three to four weeks after infection, which originates at the site of inoculation (Figure 12.1a,b; Table 12.1). Chancres are more frequent in the ano-genital region; however, extragenital locations have been reported in 12–14% of cases with 40–75% occurring in the mouth [5, 6, 9]. After eight to nine weeks, the chancre usually regresses, even without treatment.

The secondary stage is the result of dissemination of the organisms. It develops eight to nine weeks after the appearance of primary lesion. The lesions may arise before the chancre has resolved completely. Oral manifestations are polymorphous, the most common being mucous patches (Figures 12.2a,b and 12.3; Table 12.1) [9]. Spontaneous resolution of the lesions usually occurs within 3–12 weeks [5, 13]. Oral and pharyngeal manifestations can occur in approximately 30% of patients with secondary syphilis [14].

After the secondary stage, patients enter a period known as latent syphilis, in which the patient does not show clinical signs and symptoms of infection. Tertiary syphilis can occur 10 or more years after the onset of infection, affecting approximately 30–40% of patients who did not receive treatment in the primary, secondary or the latent stages of the disease [5]. Tertiary stage is characterised by the occurrence of granulomatous nodules,

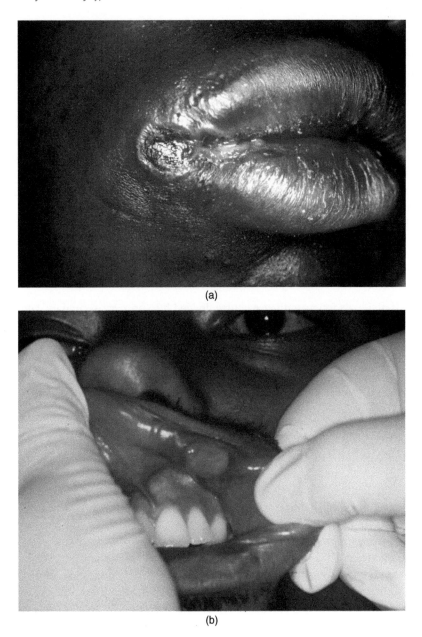

(a)

(b)

Figure 12.1 (a) Primary syphilis – oral chancre. This woman with primary syphilis developed an oral chancre at the right corner of her mouth. Syphilitic chancres are typically round, firm and painless. Source: Reproduced with permission from National STD curriculum University of Washington. (b) Primary syphilis. Chancre characterised by a raised indurated ulcer with erythematous halo and base covered with necrotic material. *Treponema pallidum* were identified in the sample collected from the lesion. Source: Courtesy of Professor Luiz Carlos Moreira Brazil.

Table 12.1 Oral manifestations of acquired syphilis and laboratory diagnosis at different stages of the disease [10–13].

Primary syphilis	
Oral manifestations	**Laboratory diagnosis**
• Oral chancres are seen most commonly on the lip, but other sites include the tongue, palate, gingiva and tonsils. • The lesion begins as a firm nodule. The surface breaks down after a few days, leaving a rounded ulcer with well-defined and regular margins, indurated and clean base, located in the inoculation area (Figure 12.1a, b). • Intraoral chancres are usually slightly painful. • Regional lymph nodes become enlarged, firm and painless with a rubbery consistency. • Oral chancres are highly infective, and treatment is most effective at this stage. • Erosive lesions or ulcerations covered with yellowish serous fluid associated with inflammatory lymphadenopathy in the anterior cervical region, involving the submandibular and submental chains. • The involvement of the palate is characterised by edema, erythema and displacement of the uvula and anterior tonsillar pillar. • In the tongue, especially on the dorsal surface, the lesion presents as an ulcer with firm and hard consistency to palpation, with the inflammed foliaceous lingual papillae.	• Direct search for *T. pallidum* in lesion samples, lymph node aspirate and/or biopsy material. Other tests include dark-field microscopy and/or nucleic acid amplification test (NAAT) from ulcer swabs. • A biopsy may show non-specific inflammation but sometimes there is conspicuous perivascular inflammation with predominance of plasma cells and psoriasiform epithelial hyperplasia. Diagnosis depends on detection of *Treponema pallidum* by Warthin–Starry staining, by immunohistochemistry or by dark-field illumination of a smear from the chancre. • Antibodies begin to appear in the bloodstream about 7–10 days after chancre appears. • Serological reactions are negative at first. When there is no reactivity, the test should be repeated after approximately 30 days to confirm the infection. • When there is a history of treated syphilis, the laboratory diagnosis must consider the titre found in the quantitative non-treponemal test.
Secondary syphilis	
• The presence or history of asymptomatic pinkish macules distributed on the trunk is a useful aid to diagnosis. • Oral lesions mainly affect tonsils, lateral borders of the tongue and lips. • Mucous patches are smooth-surfaced plaques that manifest a glistening, opalescent appearance (Figure 12.2a, b). • Condylomata lata: hypertrophic broad-based, papules with flat moist tops (Figure 12.3). • Split papules at the commissure and a maculopapular rash may be present • Oral lesions contain many spirochetes and saliva is highly infective.	• All tests that detect treponemal antibodies are reactive and non-treponemal quantitative tests have high titres. • A biopsy may show non-specific inflammation but sometimes there is conspicuous perivascular inflammation with predominance of plasma cells and psoriasiform epithelial hyperplasia. Diagnosis depends on detection of *T. pallidum* by Warthin–Starry staining, by immunohistochemistry or by dark-field illumination of a smear from the chancre. • After secondary syphilis treatment, treponemal tests may remain reactive throughout a lifetime, and non-treponemal tests can become non-reactive or remain reactive indefinitely at low rates.

(Continued)

Table 12.1 (Continued)

Oral manifestations	Laboratory diagnosis
Latent syphilis early and late	
• Absence of signs or symptoms	• All tests that detect antibodies remain reactive.
	• Decrease in titers in quantitative non-treponemal tests.
Tertiary syphilis	
• Gumma occurs mostly in the midline of the palate or dorsum of the tongue. Clinically, it begins as a swelling, sometimes with a yellowish centre, which undergoes necrosis, leaving a painless indolent deep ulcer. The ulcer is rounded, with soft, punched-out edges. The base is depressed and pale in appearance. When the palate is involved, ulceration can cause perforation toward the nasal cavity or maxillary sinus (Figure 12.4). The lesion is not infectious.	• Tests that detect antibodies are usually reactive, particularly treponemal tests.
	• Antibody titres on non-treponemal tests tend to be low and may rarely be negative.
	• Ideally, for the diagnosis of tertiary syphilis, samples from organs with suspected pathogen activity should be investigated.
• Occasional cases of syphilitic osteomyelitis involving the mandible and maxilla have been described. This condition represents a gummatous involvement of bone with extensive necrosis.	• For people with neurological symptoms, venereal disease research laboratory (VDRL) is the recommended test for cerebrospinal fluid (CSF) testing.
• The tongue may be diffusely involved becoming enlarged and lobulated (interstitial glossitis). Atrophy and loss of the papillae may be observed on the dorsum of the tongue (luetic glossitis). Leukoplakia is frequently present.	

psoriasiform plaques and gummas (Table 12.1). Tertiary syphilis is less common today, perhaps owing to the wide use of antibiotics.

Oral Manifestations

Oral manifestations of syphilis occur in primary, secondary and tertiary stages of the disease. These include appearance of chancre in the primary stage, mucous patches in the secondary stage and gumma in the tertiary stage. Detailed description of these lesions is provided in Table 12.1.

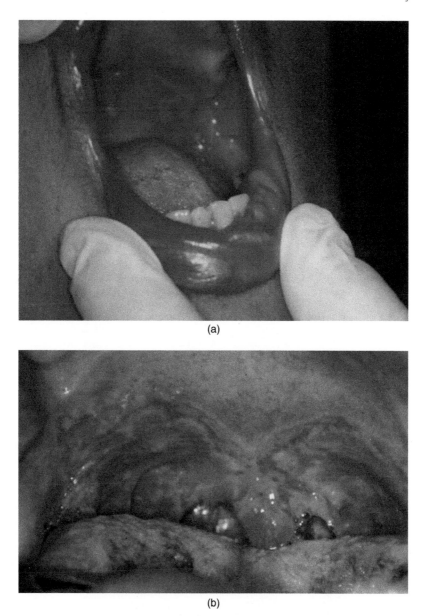

(a)

(b)

Figure 12.2 (a) Secondary syphilis showing mucous patches surrounded by erythematous halo on the lower lip, and hard and soft palates. (b) Secondary syphilis showing opal white patches with irregular edges in the soft palate and oropharynx. Source: Courtesy of Professor Luiz Carlos Moreira Brazil.

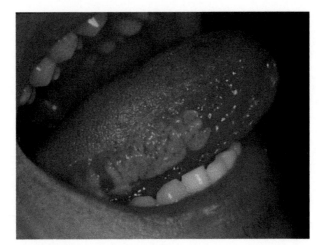

Figure 12.3 Secondary syphilis. Syphilitic condyloma (condyloma latum) showing irregular, elevated white necrotic patches with wrinkled surface on the lateral border of the tongue. Source: Courtesy of Professor Luiz Carlos Moreira Brazil.

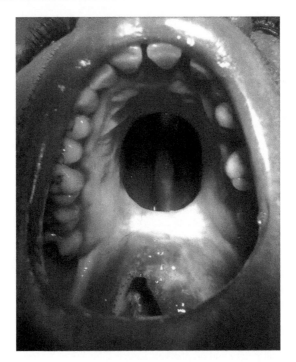

Figure 12.4 Tertiary syphilis. Intraoral view showing gummatous perforations in the hard and soft palates [17]. Source: By kind permission Dr. F Titinchi Department of Maxillofacial and Oral Surgery, Faculty of Dentistry, University of the Western Cape, Cape Town, South Africa. Courtesy of Dr. Fadi. Titinchi, University of the Western Cape, Cape Town, South Africa.

Congenital Syphilis (CS)

The three pathognomonic diagnostic features of CS, known as Hutchinson's triad, are Hutchinson's teeth (Figure 12.5a, b; Table 12.2), ocular interstitial keratitis and eighth nerve deafness [14]. However, some patients exhibit all three features. In addition to Hutchinson's teeth, a number of other oral alterations may be seen such as short maxilla, open bite, 'Gothic palate' (high-arched palate), mulberry molars and relative mandibular prognathism [14, 15].

According to Putkonen (1962), who investigated 235 patients with congenital syphilis, 45% had Hutchinson's incisors and 22% presented with Moon's molars (Table 12.2). However, only 12% showed cortical thickening related to periostitis [14]. Therefore, dental findings of syphilis have a diagnostic advantage over bone deformities. Hypoplastic changes appear in calcifying structures after the first year of life, as permanent incisors and first molars, causing enamel alteration and affecting tooth formation for limited periods. The deciduous teeth are minimally affected. Usually, these teeth are well developed by the time the spirochetes invade the developing dental tissues. The infection may result in the complete failure of development of a permanent tooth or the production of malformed teeth (Figure 12.5c; Table 12.2) [12, 13]. Oral soft tissue features in CS may include perioral fissuring (rhagades).

Differential Diagnosis

Primary syphilis is characterised by the presence of an oral chancre, which is usually an indurated ulcer with raised borders mimicking ulcer of squamous cell carcinoma [2]. Major aphthous ulcers can also be large and indurated but heal when treated with corticosteroids. Chronic granulomatous infections may be ulcerated, but they do not resolve spontaneously; tuberculosis usually causes a single indurated ulcer in the tongue, while deep mycoses are characterised by multiple non-healing, slightly raised ulcerations in the oral cavity [5, 13, 14, 18].

Oral lesions of secondary syphilis are of two basic types: a macular and papular eruption or the mucous patches, the latter being the most common. The differential diagnosis of oral mucous patches of secondary syphilis would include conditions such as chronic hyperplastic candidiasis, oral leukoplakia, oral hairy leukoplakia and plaque-form lichen planus [13]. Clinically, the secondary stage is extremely diverse [2]; however, the diagnosis can always be confirmed by serology.

The characteristic lesion of tertiary syphilis is the gumma, which occur mostly in the midline of the palate or the midline of the dorsum of the tongue [7, 17]. Clinically, gummatous ulceration of the palate may mimic traumatic ulcers such as physical injury with a foreign object, immune-mediated or malignant diseases, cocaine-related chemical injury, necrotizing sialometaplasia, eosinophilic granulomatosis with polyangiitis, sarcoidosis, mucoepidermoid carcinoma, adenoid cystic carcinoma, natural killer (NK)/T-cell lymphoma nasal type, olfactory neuroblastoma and sinonasal undifferentiated carcinoma. Additionally, other infections may be associated with palatal ulceration and perforation such as zygomycosis, aspergillosis, histoplasmosis, tuberculosis, leprosy, rhino scleroderma and leishmaniasis.

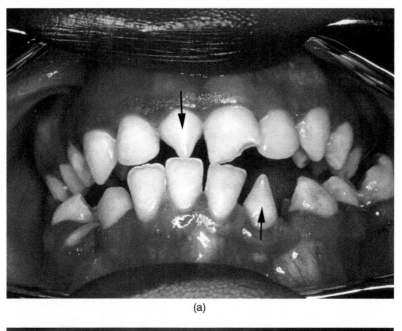

(a)

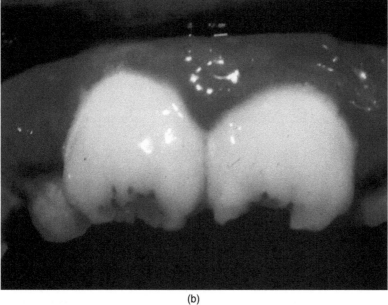

(b)

Figure 12.5 (a) Congenital syphilis. Hutchinson's teeth. This photograph demonstrates the triangular-shaped deformity of an upper central incisor (top arrow) and a lower lateral incisor (bottom arrow) dentition within the oral cavity of a person with a history of congenital syphilis. These dental abnormalities are known as Hutchinson's incisors. (b) Congenital syphilis. Hutchinson's maxillary incisors showing teeth shaped in the form of the head of a screwdriver.

(Continued)

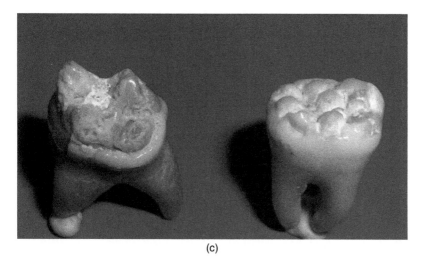

(c)

Figure 12.5 (Cont'd) (c) Congenital syphilis – Mulberry molars (Fournier's molars) with globular appearance observed on the occlusal surface of first permanent molars.

Table 12.2 Dental defects in congenital syphilis.

- Hutchinson's incisors: The upper central incisors are most commonly affected and present a 'screwdriver'-shaped or notched incisal edge. The tooth tends to be short and narrow, presenting a bulbous crown, described as 'barrel shaped' (Figure 12.5a,b).
- Mulberry molars (Fournier's molars): First permanent molar defect highly suggestive of prenatal syphilis. The teeth are smaller in size than normal. The occlusal surfaces are dome-shaped, with improperly developed cusps, producing a mulberry-like surface. These teeth are poorly enamelised and are highly prone to decay (Figure 12.5c).
- Moon's molars or bud molars: The crowns are widest at the base and narrowest at the cusps, have no grooves running around the cusps and the crown surface is smooth.
- Syphilitic canine: The maxillary and mandibular canines are smaller than normal and do not have an identifiable canine mesial crest, a distal accessory ridge or dental tubercle.

Source: Putkonen [15].

Histopathology of Oral Lesions

Descriptions of the histopathological features of oral syphilis are scarce. Oral lesions of primary and secondary syphilis show plasma cell infiltration. Overlying epithelium may show hyperplasia or pseudocarcinomatous hyperplasia, but these features are not common. Endarteritis is common. The tertiary lesion shows features of chronic granulomatous inflammation with Langerhans-type giant cells. The inflammatory process in early nodular lesions does not show necrosis. The Warthin–Starry (WS) method (silver impregnation technique) of staining of paraffin-fixed sections may reveal the presence of *T. pallidum* in the surface epithelium, intercellular spaces adjacent to blood vessels, macrophages, endothelial cells and plasma cells [18].

Diagnosis

The diagnosis of syphilis including oral manifestations of the disease is based on a full sexual history, clinical examination, serological tests and histopathological examination [8]. It is important to obtain a personal sexual history to understand the likelihood of a person having an STI. The person should be asked about their sexual practices, including oral sex, use of sex toys, and whether there is any protection (i.e. condoms) and whether the sexual partner is regular or casual, and if there is more than one sexual partner. After obtaining a sexual history, the professional needs to make patients feel comfortable to discuss personal and intimate issues about their sex life. Strategies to help patients to feel comfortable in answering sexual health questions include: normalizing by sharing with the patient that you ask these questions to all your patients, discussing that you will use the information gained to better care for the patient, and sharing that the answers are confidential and will not be shared with anyone outside of the healthcare team.

A careful physical examination and the results of laboratory tests complement the clinical investigation. The tests used to diagnose syphilis are divided into two categories: direct examinations and immunological tests. Direct examinations investigate the presence of *T. pallidum* in samples collected directly from primary and secondary lesions or by the nucleic acid amplification test (NAAT). The survey is carried out on stained material or by dark-field microscopy. By immunohistochemistry, the antibody anti-*T. pallidum* may be useful. A positive test indicates active infection; however, a negative test may result from an insufficient number of the microorganisms in the sample studied.

Serological tests, the most used in clinical practice, are subdivided into two classes: treponemal and non-treponemal, and investigate the presence of antibodies in whole blood, serum or plasma samples [2, 8].

Non-treponemal tests are quantifiable and detect non-specific antibodies to *T. pallidum* antigens. When the result is reactive, the sample is diluted in order to obtain a titration of these antibodies. Any titration should be investigated as a case of syphilis. Titers lower than 1:4 can be found in recent and late stages of the infection and may persist for months or years. In some cases, even after treatment, a low titre may remain [8]. This event can be temporary or persistent and is called serofast status. Serial non-treponemal tests are performed to monitor response to treatment.

Treponemal tests are the first to become reactive. They can remain reactive for life and, therefore, are not indicated for monitoring the response to treatment. The laboratory investigation of syphilis should start with a treponemal test, preferably the rapid test, due to its greater sensitivity and quick turn-around time in a field setting. The interpretation of the tests depends on the combination used between the treponemal and non-treponemal tests.

Pregnant women should be tested for syphilis at the first prenatal visit (ideally in the first trimester), at the beginning of the third trimester and at admission for childbirth, in case of miscarriage, stillbirth, history of exposure to risk or sexual violence. Clinical and laboratory monitoring with the non-treponemal test should be performed monthly during pregnancy. After delivery, this follow-up is performed quarterly until the 12th month.

The laboratory investigation of syphilis should start with a treponemal test, preferably the rapid test, due to its greater sensitivity. The interpretation of the tests depends on the combination used between the treponemal and non-treponemal tests.

Treatment, Prognosis and Complications

Benzathine penicillin G or aqueous *Procaine penicillin G* remains the drug of choice for all forms of syphilis. Oral *doxycycline* 100 mg orally twice for 14 days is effective against *T. pallidum*. This is used for patients who are allergic to penicillin. These regimens are valid for primary, secondary and early latent syphilis. In syphilis of more than 1 year's duration (or unknown duration), treatment is given for 28 days in the same dosage. Both ceftriaxone and azithromycin are effective in the treatment of early syphilis. A problem with azithromycin is increasing resistance of *T. pallidum*. If left untreated, the disease can progress to severe systemic complications several years after the initial infection.

A patient with a confirmed diagnosis of syphilis should be treated immediately after a confirmed diagnosis [8]. Serologic response to treatment should be evident by 6 months in early syphilis and 12–24 months for latent syphilis [9].

Post-treatment monitoring with non-treponemal testing should be performed to determine adequate serologic response [9]. Treatment success is observed with a decrease in the titration in two dilutions of the non-treponemal tests within three months and four dilutions within six months, with evolution to seroreversion (non-reactive non-treponemal test). Clinical follow-up should continue after treatment to monitor for possible reactivation or reinfection.

If left untreated, syphilis can progress to severe systemic complications several years after the initial infection. Screening for syphilis should be part of the follow-up of every pregnant woman to avoid miscarriage, prematurity, low birth weight, stillbirth and early or late clinical manifestations of CS [9].

The Jarisch–Herxheimer reaction is an episode that can occur within the first 24 hours after starting treatment with penicillin, especially in primary and secondary syphilis. It manifests through exacerbation of skin lesions, with erythema, pain or itching, general malaise, fever, headache and arthralgia, which spontaneously regress after 12–24 hours [9].

Referral/Prevention/Patient Education

In some cases, syphilis patients should be referred for treatment in a hospital or a specialist care environment. Syphilis requires the participation of numerous professionals in its fight involving healthcare workers including dentists, making this group the main front line. The use of male and female condoms is recommended in the prevention of STIs.

References

1 Hook, E.W. 3rd. (2017). Syphilis. *Lancet* 389 (10078): 1550–1557.
2 Andrade, R.S., Freitas, E.M., Rocha, B.A. et al. (2018). Oral findings in secondary syphilis. *Med. Oral Patol. Oral Cir. Bucal* 23 (2): e138–e143.
3 Peeling, R.W., Mabey, D., Kamb, M.L. et al. (2017). Syphilis. *Nat. Rev. Dis. Primers* 12 (3): 17073.

4 Ficarra, G. and Carlos, R. (2009). Syphilis: the renaissance of an old disease with oral implications. *Head Neck Pathol.* 3 (3): 195–206. https://doi.org/10.1007/s12105-009-0127-0.

5 Smith, M.H., Vargo, R.J., Bilodeau, E.A. et al. (2021). Oral manifestations of syphilis: a review of the clinical and histopathologic characteristics of a reemerging entity with report of 19. *New Cases Head Neck Pathol.* 15 (3): 787–795. Published online 2021 Jan 18.

6 Yu, X. and Zheng, H. (2016). Syphilitic chancre of the lips transmitted by kissing. *Medicine* 95: 1–2.

7 Queirós, C. and Costa, J.B. (2019). Oral transmission of sexually Transmissable infections: a narrative review. *Acta Med. Port.* 32 (12): 776–781.

8 Workowski, K.A. and Bolan, G.A. (2015). Centers for Diseasee Control and Prevention. Sexually Transmitted Diseases Treatment Guidelines. *MMWR Recomm Rep* Jun 5;64(RR-03):1–137. Erratum in: MMWR Recomm Rep. 2015 Aug 28;64(33):924.

9 Singh, A.E. and Romanowski, B. (1999). Syphilis: review with emphasis on clinical, epidemiologic, and some biologic features. *Clin. Microbiol. Rev.* 12 (2): 187–209.

10 Centres for Disease Control and Prevention (2021). Ways HIV Can Be Transmitted/HIV Transmission. https://www.cdc.gov/hiv/basics/hiv-transmission/ways-people-get-hiv.html

11 Copen, C.E., Chandra, A., and Febo-Vazquez, I. (2016). Sexual behavior, sexual attraction, and sexual orientation among adults aged 18–44 in the United States: data from the 2011–2013 National Survey of Family Growth. *Natl. Health Stat. Rep.* 88: 1–14. PMID: 26766410.

12 Lautenschlager, S. (2006). Diagnosis of syphilis: clinical and laboratory problems. *J. Dtsch. Dermatol. Ges.* 4 (12): 1058–1075. https://doi.org/10.1111/j.1610-0387.2006.06072.x.

13 Fitzpatrick, S.G., Cohen, D.M., and Clark, A.N. (2019). SPECIAL ISSUE: colors and textures, a review of oral mucosal entities ulcerated lesions of the oral mucosa: clinical and histologic review. *Head Neck Pathol.* 13: 91–102.

14 Leão, J.C., Gueiros, L.A., and Porter, S.R. (2006). Oral manifestations of syphilis. *Clinics* 61 (2): 161–166.

15 Putkonen, T. (1962). Dental changes in congenital syphilis. Relationship to other syphilitic stigmata. *Acta Derm. Venereol.* 42: 44–62.

16 Pessoa, L. and Galvão, V. (2011). Clinical aspects of congenital syphilis with Hutchinson's triad. *BMJ Case Rep.* 2011: bcr1120115130. https://doi.org/10.1136/bcr.11.2011.5130.

17 Salazar, J.F.T. and Ortega, D.R. (2017). Signos dentales de la sífilis congénita / Dental signs of congenital syphilis. *Rev. ADM* 74 (6): 286–292.

18 Leuci, S., Martina, S., Adamo, D. et al. (2012). Oral syphilis: a retrospective analysis of 12 cases and a review of the literature. *Oral Dis.* 19 (8): 738–746.

19 Titinchi, F., Behardien, N., Morkel, J., and Opperman, J. (2020). Perforation of the palate – a report of two syphilitic Gumma cases. *S. Afr. Dent. J.* 75 (6): 311–315. https://dx.doi.org/10.17159/2519-0105/2020/v75no6a4.

20 Barrett, A.W., Villarroel Dorrego, M., Hodgson, T.A. et al. (2004). The histopathology of syphilis of the oral mucosa. *J. Oral Pathol. Med.* 33 (5): 286–291.

13

Oral Manifestations of Gonorrhoea

Anura Ariyawardana[1,2,3]

[1]*School of Medicine and Dentistry, Griffith University, Gold Coast, Australia*
[2]*College of Medicine and Dentistry, James Cook University, Cairns, Australia*
[3]*Clinical Principal, Metro South Oral Health, Queensland Health, Brisbane, Australia*

Introduction

Gonorrhoea is a sexually transmitted disease caused by a Gram-negative diplococcus, *Neisseria gonorrhoeae. This* organism is pathogenic exclusively for humans and is usually localised in the urogenital, oral–pharyngeal and anal mucous membranes [1, 2]. Globally, gonorrhoea has become a significant threat to human health especially due to the rapid development of anti-microbial resistance experienced in the recent years [1]. According to the World Health Organization (WHO) estimates in 2016, nearly 87 million individuals globally acquired gonorrhoea infection with incidence rates of 20 and 26 per 1000 women and men, respectively [3].

Gonorrhoea readily transmits through unprotected sex. It has been estimated that probability of male-to-female transmission is ~50% while female-to-male transmission is ~20% per sex act [2]. Based on mathematical modelling, Hui et al. reported estimated probabilities of transmission during unprotected oral (63% urethral-to-pharyngeal and 9% pharyngeal-to-urethral cases) and anal sex (84% urethral-to-rectal and 2% rectal to-urethral cases) [4]. This chapter describes pathogenesis, clinical features and management of oral manifestations of gonorrhoea. Detailed description of gonorrhoea can be found in Chapter 1.

Epidemiology of Oropharyngeal Gonorrhoea

Chan and colleagues reviewed the literature describing prevalence of extra genital sexually transmitted diseases, which include oropharyngeal gonorrhoea [5]. This study reported the prevalence of extra genital infections in women, men who have sex with men (MSM), and men who have sex only with women (MSW) (Tables 13.1–13.3). The prevalence of oropharyngeal gonorrhoea among women was reported to vary from 0.3 to 29.6% (Table 13.1).

Sexually Transmissible Oral Diseases, First Edition.
Edited by S.R. Prabhu, Nicholas van Wagoner, Jeff Hill and Shailendra Sawleshwarkar.
© 2023 John Wiley & Sons Ltd. Published 2023 by John Wiley & Sons Ltd.

Table 13.1 Prevalence of pharyngeal gonorrhoea among women.

Author, Year	Country	Sample size	Prevalence (%)
Linhart et al., 2008	Israel	300	9.0
Giannini et al., 2019	USA	1949	2.5–6.8
Peters et al., 2011	Netherlands	4299	0.8
Koedijk et al., 2012	Netherlands	207134	1.2
Mayer et al., 2012	USA	119	2.0
Diaz et al., 2013	Spain	318	29.6
Shaw et al., 2013	UK	2808	0.3
Van Liere et al., 2013	Netherlands	1321	2.3
Jenkins et al., 2014	USA	301	0.70
Van Liere et al., 2014	Netherlands	1321	2.3
Danby et al., 2016	USA	175	2.3
Muijrers et al., 2015	Netherlands	7419	2.7
Garner et al., 2015	UK	649	0.6
Trebach et al., 2015	USA	4402	2.1
Bachman et al., 2010	USA	99	8.20

Source: Adapted from Chan et al. [5].

Among men who had sex with men, oro-pharyngeal gonorrhoea was reported to be 0.5–16.5% (Table 13.2). Men who had sex with women was reported to have oro-pharyngeal infections varying from 1.2–15.5 % (Tables 13.3).

Transmission

Behavioural changes in sexual practices, taken place over the years, have made individuals more vulnerable to oral transmission of gonorrhoea [6]. The epithelium of the uterine cervix, urethra and the transitional epithelium of the oropharynx and rectum are common entry points for gonococcal infection. Although, fellatio has generally been regarded as the sole means of transmission of gonorrhoea to the oropharyngeal tissues, colonisation has also been identified among people with no such sexual practices [7]. A recent study carried out in Australia reported that oropharyngeal gonorrhoea infection was common among heterosexual women and heterosexual men with untreated urogenital gonorrhoea [8]. Moreover, gonorrhoea can also be transmitted in the absence of urogenital infection [9]. Oropharyngeal gonorrhoea is mostly asymptomatic and hence the transmission through oropharyngeal sex practices is highly likely [7, 10, 11]. Transmission via saliva from an infected partner with oropharyngeal gonorrhoea through deep kissing has also been considered [11].

Table 13.2 Prevalence of pharyngeal gonorrhoea among men who had sex with men.

Author, Year	Country	Sample size	Prevalence (%)
Tabet et al., 1998	USA	578	0.70
Kent et al., 2005	USA	6434	9.2
Morris et al., 2006	USA	2475	5.5
Benn et al., 2007	UK	613	7.3
Alexander et al., 2008	UK	272	6.5
Gunn et al., 2008	USA	7333	4.0
Rieg et al., 2008	USA	212	3.3
Annan et al., 2009	UK	3076	1.3
Baker et al., 2009	USA	147	2.8
Klausner et al., 2009	USA	17599	5.3
Mimiaga et al., 2009	USA	21927	1.9
Ota et al., 2009	Canada	248	8.1
Templeton et al., 2010	Australia	1427	0.6
Marcus et al., 2011	USA	3398	5.0
Peters et al., 2011	Netherlands	1455	4.2
Soni and White	UK	634	3.9
Vodstrcil et al., 2011	Australia	15460	1.8
Koedijk et al., 2012	Netherlands	69506	3.90
Mayer et al., 2012	USA	365	3.0
Park et al., 2012	USA	12454	5.8
Pinsky et al., 2012	USA	200	3.5
Diaz et al., 2013	Spain	1320	5.2
Jimenez et al., 2013	Spain	264	9.5
Sexton et al., 2013	USA	374	9.3
Barbee et al., 2014	USA	3034	6.5
Viule et al., 2014	Germany	2247	5.5
Keaveney et al., 2014	Ireland	121	3.3
Patton et al., 2014	USA	21994	7.9
Van Liere et al., 2014	Netherlands	2436	3.4
Chow et al., 2015	Australia	12876	1.7
Danby et al., 2016	USA	224	16.5
Muijrers et al., 2015	Netherlands	2349	3.4
Garner et al., 2015	UK	365	5.2
Tongtoyai et al., 2015	Thailand	1744	0.5
Trebach et al., 2015	USA	769	11.0
Bachman et al., 2010	USA	297	8.3

Source: Adapted from Chan et al. [5].

Table 13.3 Prevalence of pharyngeal gonorrhoea among men who had sex with women.

Author, Year	Country	Sample size	Prevalence (%)
Chan et al., 2012	USA	21 379	3.4
Rodriguez-Hart et al., 2012	USA	168	1.2
Jenkins et al., 2014	USA	192	2.1
Oda et al., 2014	Japan	225	2.2
Patterson et al., 2014	USA	316	15.5

Source: Adapted from Chan et al. [5].

Pathogenesis

The susceptibility for *N. gonorrhoeae* infection depends on the tissue characteristics. The columnar epithelium of the cervix and urethra and transitional epithelium of the oropharynx and rectum are common entry points for gonococcal infection. The stratified squamous epithelium of the oral cavity appears more resistant infection [6]. Upon transmission, *N. gonorrhoeae* colonises on the oral mucosa and expresses a range of factors that enable the organism to replicate and establish in the oropharyngeal environment while some factors help evade the host immune system [12].

Pharyngeal Colonisation

In a case–control study, Javanbakht and colleagues reported 28% pharyngeal-only infections among 64 cases while 27% had both urogenital and pharyngeal infections indicating the risk of gonorrhoea transmission through oropharyngeal sex practices [13]. Another Australian clinical study found pharyngeal gonorrhoea among 9/33 (27.3%) heterosexual female cases. The study indicated pharyngeal colonisation among females is an important reservoir for transmission of the infection to heterosexual males [14]. Pathogenic mechanism, however, is not very well understood [7, 12].

Oral Manifestations

Oropharyngeal gonorrhoea is generally asymptomatic [15]. However, some may have mild-to-moderate sore throat. Tonsilitis typically demonstrates oedema, erythema with accompanying scattered small punctate pustules. Oral features include gingivitis, glossitis, multiple oral mucosal ulcers, erythema and white pseudomembrane (Figure 13.1). Cervical lymphadenopathy can accompany oropharyngeal gonorrhoea [16]. However, the lesions of oral gonorrhoea are not specific and may mimic a wide array of oral diseases including herpes simplex infections, erythema multiforme and vesiculo-bullous disorders [17, 18].

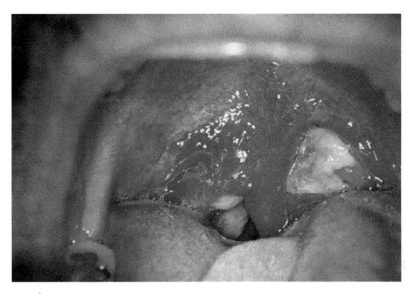

Figure 13.1 Gonococcal stomatitis. Note mucosal erythema and pseudomembrane of the soft palate. Source: Reproduced with permission from Professor Luiz Carlos Moreira, Brazil.

Diagnosis

Diagnosis of oral and pharyngeal gonorrhoea is difficult to some extent due to the lack of symptoms and non-specific nature of the manifestations [18]. However, detailed history of the sexual contacts might be of help in ascertaining the cause of the infection.

Nucleic acid amplification tests (NAATs) can detect *N. gonorrhoeae*-specific DNA or RNA. However, this is considered less sensitive in diagnosing extra genital gonorrhoea possibly due to the colonisation of these sites with a wide range of other organisms, including other *Neisseria* species, likely interfering with *N. gonorrhoeae* isolation. Further, sometimes this technique is unable to determine the antibiotic sensitivity. Therefore, culture is the preferred diagnostic method [5, 16]; see Chapter 3 for other details.

Treatment

Treatment of gonorrhoea is difficult to attribute to the ability of the organism to develop antibiotic resistance. Multi-drug resistance including sulphonamides, penicillins, tetracyclines, macrolides, fluoroquinolones, and cephalosporins are of a concern [15].

Therapeutic strategies recommended for oral–gonococcal infection are based on oral *cefixime* or intramuscular *ceftriaxone*. However, the patients diagnosed with a sexually transmitted disease would often have more than one types of infection [18]. It is recommended to refer the patients to relevant specialists to take care of any likely genital infection and general advice on prevention through sexual transmission. Oropharyngeal gonorrhoea is difficult to treat and a test of cure is recommended.

References

1 Kinga, R., Piotr, P., and Halina, P.-S. (2019). Gonorrhoea – current threat? Epidemiological analysis of gonococcal infections. *Journal Educ. Health and Sport* 9 (9): 406–414.

2 Kirkcaldy, R.D., Weston, E., Segurado, A.C., and Hug, G. (2019). Epidemiology of gonorrhoea: a global perspective. *Sex. Health* 16: 401–411.

3 Rowley, J., Hoorn, S.V., Korenromp, E. et al. (2019). Chlamydia, gonorrhoea, trichomoniasis and syphilis: global prevalence and incidence estimates, 2016. *Bull. World Health Organ.* 97: 548–562P.

4 Hui, B., Fairley, C.K., Chen, M. et al. (2015). Oral and anal sex are key to sustaining gonorrhea at endemic levels in MSM populations: a mathematical model. *Sex. Transm. Infect.* 91 (5): 365–369.

5 Chan, P.A., Robinette, A., Montgomery, M. et al. (2016). Extragenital infections caused by *Chlamydia trachomatis* and *Neisseria gonorrhoeae*: a review of the literature. *Infect. Dis. Obstet. Gynecol.* 2016: 5758387. https://doi.org/10.1155/2016/5758387.

6 Queiros, C. and da Costa, J.B. (2019). Oral transmission of sexually Transmissable infections: a narrative review. *Acta Med. Port.* 32 (12): 776–781.

7 Osborne, N.G. and Grubin, L. (1979). Colonozation of the pharynx with *Neisseria gonorrhoea*: experience in a clinic for sexually transmitted diseases. *Sex. Transm. Dis.* 253–256.

8 Allen, C., Fairley, C.K., Chen, M.Y. et al. (2021). Oropharyngeal gonorrhoea infections among heterosexual women and heterosexual men with urogenital gonorrhoea attending a sexual health clinic in Melbourne, Australia. *Clinical Microbiology and Infection* 27 (12): P1799–P1804. https://doi.org/10.1016/j.cmi.2021.03.033.

9 Cornelisse, W.J., Bradshaw, C.S., Chow, E.P.F. et al. (2019). Oropharyngeal gonorrhea in absence of urogenital gonorrhea in sexual network of male and female participants, Australia, 2018. *Emerg. Infect. Dis.* 25 (7): 1373–1376.

10 Fairley, C.K., Cornelisse, V.J., Hocking, J.S., and Chow, E.P.F. (2019). Models of gonorrhoea transmission from the mouth and saliva. *Lancet Infect. Dis.* 19 (10): e360–e366. https://doi.org/10.1016/S1473-3099(19)30304-4.

11 Fairley, C.K., Hocking, J.S., Zhang, L., and Chow, E.P. (2017). Frequent transmission of gonorrhea in men who have sex with men. *Emerg. Infect. Dis.* 23 (1): 102–104. https://doi.org/10.3201/eid2301.161205.

12 Quillin, S.J. and Seifert, H.S. (2018). *Neisseria gonorrhoeae* host adaptation and pathogenesis. *Nature Reviews Microbiology* 16: 226–240. https://doi.org/10.1038/nrmicro.2017.169.

13 Javanbakht, M., Westmoreland, D., and Gorbach, P. (2018). Factors associated with pharyngeal gonorrhea in young people: implications for prevention. *Sex. Transm. Dis.* 45 (9): 588–593. https://doi.org/10.1097/OLQ.0000000000000822.

14 Lusk, M.J., Uddin, R.N.N., Lahra, M.M. et al. (2013). Pharyngeal Gonorrhoea in women: an important reservoir for increasing *Neisseria gonorrhoea* prevalence in urban Australian heterosexuals? *J. Sex. Transm. Dis.* Article ID 967471, https://doi.org/10.1155/2013/967471.

15 Morgan, M.K. and Decker, C.F. (2016). Gonorrhoea. *Dis. Mon.* 62: 260–268.

16 Neville, B.W., Damm, D.D., Allen, C.M., and Chi, A.C. (2016). *Oral and Maxillofacial Pathology*, 4e, 174–176. St Louis, Missouri: Elsevier.

17 Bruce, A.J. and Rogers, R.S. (2004). Oral manifestations of sexually transmitted diseases. *Clin. Dermatol.* 22: 520–527.

18 Fernández-López, C. and Morales-Angulo, C. (2017). Otorhinolaryngology manifestations secondary to oral sex. *Acta Otorrinolaringol. Esp.* 68 (3): 169–180. https://doi.org/10.1016/j.otoeng.2016.04.014.

14

Oral Herpes Simplex Virus Infections

Jeremy Lau and Ramesh Balasubramaniam

Oral Medicine, University of Western Australia Dental School, Perth, Australia

Introduction

There is a wide array of viral infections that can affect the oral cavity and associated structures. Some more common viruses include human herpes virus (HSV), human papillomavirus, human immunodeficiency virus and Epstein Barr virus. Human herpes viruses are classified into three subfamilies, which are alpha beta, and gamma subfamilies. The alpha subfamily includes HSV type 1 (HSV-1), and HSV type 2 (HSV-2), and varicella zoster virus (VZV). This chapter will focus on HSV infections (HSV-1 and HSV-2).

Most people with oral herpes get it from non-sexual contact with saliva. Though uncommon, oral herpes caused by HSV-1 can spread from the mouth to the genitals and HSV-2 infection from genitals to mouth through oral sex. Following an initial infection, HSV-1 and HSV-2 cause life long infection. Its presentation is often atypical and has the potential to be life threatening. After acquisition, it may present as oral, orofacial, genital and ocular lesions.

Epidemiology

HSV is extremely prevalent, infecting billions around the world. According to the World Health Organization, HSV-1 has a seroprevalence of 67% of the global population under the age of 50 [1].

The prevalence of infection of HSV-1 differs among continents and is reported to be the highest in Africa, at 88% of the adult population. It is estimated that there are 3.583 billion infected patients with oral HSV-1 in those up to 49 years or age [2]. HSV-2 has a seroprevalence of 13% for people aged between 15 and 49. Infection is most common in adolescence but as a life-long infection, it increases with age. HSV-2 is more common in women than men, making up to 64% of total infections in women and 36% in men. The incidence of HSV-2 infection is highest in Africa, occurring in 44% of women and 25% in men [2]. Even though HSV has a significant effect on the sexual health of millions globally, to date there

Sexually Transmissible Oral Diseases, First Edition.
Edited by S.R. Prabhu, Nicholas van Wagoner, Jeff Hill and Shailendra Sawleshwarkar.
© 2023 John Wiley & Sons Ltd. Published 2023 by John Wiley & Sons Ltd.

have been no specific studies that show the prevalence of oral HSV infection acquired exclusively through sexual activity.

Etiopathogenesis/Risk Factors/Predisposing Factors

There are various risk factors for HSV-1 infections, often different depending on whether the infection is acquired sexually or non-sexually. Risk factors for oral presentation of HSV-1 typically involve exposure to an infected individual's saliva [3]. This may occur via mouth-to-mouth contact, sharing cutlery and crockery, and sharing cosmetics. Shaving a beard with concurrent acute orolabial infection is considered a risk factor of herpetic sycosis. Herpetic sycosis is a recurrent or initial herpes simplex infection affecting primarily the hair follicles. Another form of herpes is herpes gladiatorum, in which close contact sports is considered a risk factor. Individuals, who suck thumb and bite nail, with concurrent acute orolabial HSV infection are more susceptible to herpetic whitlow [4]. In cases of herpes encephalitis, mutations of toll-like receptor (TLR-3) or UNC-93B gene are considered a significant risk factor [5]. Furthermore, skin barrier dysfunction is a major risk factor for eczema herpeticum.

Immunocompromised or immunosuppressed patients have an increased risk of developing severe or chronic HSV infections. Such patients can include transplant recipients and patients with HIV or leukaemia.

HSV-2 infection is predominantly transmitted during sex from one HSV-2 positive partner to an uninfected partner. During sexual intercourse, acquisition of HSV-2 may occur after exposure to bodily fluids, contact with genitalia, skin or sores. Sexual transmission of HSV-2 is more efficient from men to women, which explains its high incidence in women. Vertical transmission can occur during childbirth, where primary and recurrent HSV can lead to perinatal transmission and subsequent congenital HSV infection. In addition, HSV can be transmitted in the context of child sexual abuse. The presence of HSV infection in children may be an indication that sexual assault has occurred. In sexual abuse, both HSV-1 and HSV-2 can be transmitted.

Microbiology

Typically, a virus infection occurs in two stages: attachment and penetration [6]. For an infection to take place, the excreting virus must contact either mucosal surface or abraded skin. Viruses attach to host cells via cellular receptors. Viruses can penetrate cells either through fusing to the cell membrane or through a process called receptor-mediated endocytosis. When the viral genome is released, transcription and replication can then occur. Latency can be established through transport of the virus or its capsid to the dorsal root ganglia. HSV can infect any nerve. When the trigeminal ganglion is colonised, latent virus can be harboured. Once latency is established, various stimuli can reactivate disease. Triggers of reaction can include hormonal changes, infection, illness or even exposure to weather elements of cold, wind or sunlight.

The transmission of HSV is typically through contact. HSV-1 is predominantly transmitted through oral-to-oral contact but can also be transmitted via oral-to-genital contact. HSV-1 infections typically occur in the oropharyngeal mucosa. The trigeminal ganglion becomes colonised with HSV-1 and can hold the virus latent. HSV-2 is almost solely transmitted via genital contact. HSV-2 is able to replicate in the ano-genital region. Although less common, HSV-2 is also able to infect the mouth. In general, infections resulting from HSV-1 occur above the waist, whereas infections from HSV-2 typically occur below the waist [7]. However, increasing number of HSV-1 infections are reported in the genital region and overlap may occur.

HSV infections can be described as either a primary infection or a secondary infection. A primary infection occurs after an initial exposure to HSV-1 or HSV-2, where the person does not have pre-existing antibodies. Even if a person has HSV-1 antibodies, it is still possible for them to acquire an initial HSV-2 infection and vice versa. A secondary infection, also known as a recurrent infection occurs when HSV travels from the nerve to the skin or mucous membrane and causes symptoms.

Clinical Features

The majority of individuals with serological evidence of HSV-1 and HSV-2 infections commonly do not recognise that they have a current infection. Infections are often asymptomatic and do not have specific signs and symptoms. In the event where symptoms arise, primary infections have a propensity to be more severe than recurrences.

Primary HSV-1 infections typically involve the mouth. Signs and symptoms generally arise within one to two weeks exposure to the virus and may involve both systemic and oral features. Systemic features include malaise, fever, loss of appetite and lethargy. There is often bilateral cervical lymphadenopathy, and a cutaneous rash on the face for example may form [8, 9].

Oral features include vesicles and ulceration of the oral mucosa and gingiva. Ulcers on the oral mucosa and gingiva tend to be small and spherical. They may coalesce together

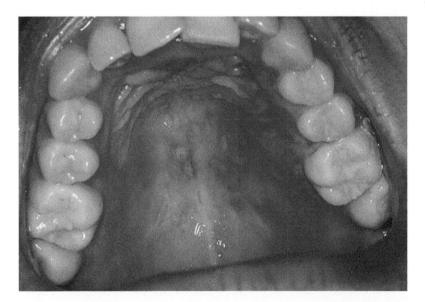

Figure 14.1 Primary herpetic gingivostomatitis. Widespread oral ulceration is noted on the patient's palate. Courtesy of Dr Alissa Jacobs, Perth Oral Medicine and Dental Sleep Centre, Perth WA, Australia.

giving rise to larger, irregular-shaped ulcers (Figure 14.1). The gingiva may appear erythematous and swollen with ulceration. Typically, signs and symptoms are self-limiting and will spontaneously resolve in 7–10 days. In individuals who are immunocompromised, resolution may take longer.

The clinical picture of primary HSV-2 is similar to HSV-1. It is thought that symptoms of HSV-2 are typically less severe, and its duration is shorter than that of HSV-1.

Recurrent HSV-1 infection commonly presents as 'cold sores' on the vermillion. It is also known as herpes labialis. It can be precipitated by a range of events such as illness, sunlight exposure, UV light, menstrual cycle, trauma, stress, oral cancer therapy or pregnancy. Its location is not restricted to the vermillion and can also present on the perioral or perinasal skin. Symptoms of herpes labialis include paraesthesia, itching and tingling often occurring prior to any signs. The typical appearance of herpes labialis includes superficial ulceration, vesiculation, erythema, blistering and pustule formation [10] (Figure 14.2). Signs and symptoms may last about five to seven days. It is common for patients to have reoccurrences at the same site, which may indicate the location of residency of HSV within the trigeminal ganglion.

Although beyond the scope of this chapter, some extra oral manifestations of herpetic infection include cutaneous herpetic, ocular and genital infections. Cutaneous infections include herpetic whitlow where patients can present with prodromal features of pain or burning sensation followed by vesicular eruption on the distal phalanges. Ocular symptoms most typically present herpetic simplex keratitis, which affects the cornea. Its

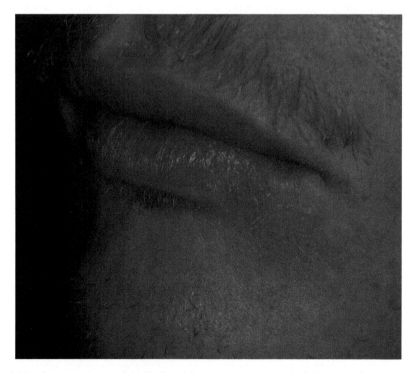

Figure 14.2 Recurrent herpes labialis. Resolving recurrent herpes labialis is noted on the patient's lower left vermillion border.

presentation can also include eyelid involvement, conjunctivitis, corneal epithelial disease, neurotrophic ulcer, corneal stromal disease, uveitis and retinitis [11]. Genital herpes, particularly from primary HSV-2, presents as extensive, bilateral genital vesicles and ulceration. Systemic symptoms of pain, fever, malaise and lymphadenopathy can also be present.

Differential Diagnosis

Recurrent Aphthous Ulcer

Oral manifestations of herpes simplex infections are often misdiagnosed as recurrent aphthous ulcers. Recurrent HSV typically involves prodromal phase with pain, itching, burning or tingling prior to vesicle or ulcer formation. Systemic effects are typically seen as a prodrome of new infection. In addition, HSV infections often present with associated erythema, whereas this is uncommon with recurrent aphthous ulcers. Recurrent aphthous ulcers may also be associated with nutritional deficiency including vitamin B12, folic acid, zinc and iron.

Viral Infections

HSV-1 and HSV-2 conditions may appear clinically similar to other viral infections particularly coxsackie viruses, herpes zoster and cytomegalovirus. Laboratory analysis is a means to distinguish between HSV infections and other viral infections.

Coxsackie Virus

Coxsackie virus may cause two conditions which involve the oral mucosa including herpangina and hand, foot and mouth diseases. Herpangina is a systemic infection common in children, where symptoms of a fever or sore throat are present. This is followed by multiple small vesicles appearing on the tonsils, uvula and palate. Unlike HSV infections, the gingiva is not typically involved. Hand, foot and mouth diseases are often seen in young children. As its name suggests, it is characterised by vesicles on the oral mucosa, hands and feet. The extra oral vesicles help distinguish it from HSV infections.

Herpes Zoster

Varicella zoster can become latent in the cranial nerves or dorsal root ganglia. When the trigeminal nerve is involved, Herpes zoster most commonly affects the ophthalmic division. In approximately 15–20% of cases, the maxillary or mandibular division of the trigeminal nerve is involved [12, 13]. Patients may experience intense pain, unilateral facial symptoms and intraoral lesions distributing along the affected nerve. Its distinct unilateral distribution and associated pain can help differentiate it from HSV infections

Acute Necrotizing Ulcerative Gingivitis

Patients with acute necrotising ulcerative gingivitis (ANUG) often present with poor oral hygiene, poor nutrition, stressors in life, and a history of smoking. The gingiva may appear to have a 'punched out', ulcerative appearance. Bleeding on probing is also likely. Unlike HSV, systematic symptoms of malaise, fever and lymphadenopathy are uncommon in ANUG.

Diagnosis/Investigations

The diagnosis of primary HSV-1 usually arises from clinical features. Especially in herpes labialis, the clinical picture is often classical; hence, it can be diagnosed from a history, signs and symptoms alone. In some cases, further investigations are warranted. Laboratory confirmation of the diagnosis is beneficial particularly when the presentation is severe, atypical or patients are immunocompromised. In addition to investigations to detect either HSV-1 or HSV-2, a full blood count may be used to rule out common causes of immunosuppression.

Investigations are used to identify HSV-1 or HSV-2 DNA through molecular means. Methods of investigation include polymerase chain reaction (PCR), cell culture, and assessment for specific immunoglobulin G (IgG) antibodies. The sample required for testing can be collected from the lesion in the perioral area. When testing for antibodies, a blood sample is taken. In rare cases, where encephalitis or meningitis is suspected, a sample of cerebrospinal fluid via a lumbar puncture can be taken.

The typical clinical method to detect HSV is via tissue culture. Cell culture is considered less expensive than other methods such as PCR. Swabs of active lesions are considered the gold standard; however, limitations of this method result from the short time frame of viral shredding.

Antibody testing assesses for immune proteins, specifically IgG, in the blood. During a response to a herpes infection, the body produces IgG antibodies. A positive antibody test indicates that there is either a current or past infection regardless of symptoms. If there is a recent HSV infection, the body may not have had sufficient time to produce antibodies; thus, it is possible to obtain a negative result even with an infection. During an acute phase, there can be greater than four times the number specific IgG antibodies in comparison to the convalescent phase. The acute phase typically occurs in the first three days, and the convalescent phase in the following two to three weeks. Furthermore, testing is able to detect and distinguish between both HSV-1 and HSV-2 antibodies.

A PCR test is used to identify HSV DNA, and is highly sensitive and specific [14]. A positive PCR test indicates that there is an active HSV infection. It can also differentiate between HSV-1 and HSV-2. Although a negative test typically indicates that HSV is not detected, it can occasionally be a false negative, particularly if the quantity of virus particles is too low to detect. In most cases, PCR testing is considered the preferred method of investigation where clinical signs are present.

Management

Management Strategies

Management of primary HSV-1 includes a symptomatic relief while the infection runs its course. Topical anti-inflammatory medication or mouthwashes may be used to reduce symptoms. Relief can also be found with topical anaesthetics such as lignocaine gel. Systemically, ibuprofen can act as an anti-inflammatory, or paracetamol can be taken as an antipyretic and analgesic. In some cases, particularly with herpes labialis, treatment is not always necessary [15]. Signs and symptoms almost always resolve in two weeks.

Table 14.1 Summary of common antiviral medications against HSV.

Medication	Class	Treatment dosage	Prophylaxis dose	Clinical indications
Acyclovir	Acyclic guanine nucleoside (false nucleotide)	Oral 200 mg five times a day	Oral 200 mg thrice a day	Treatment and prophylaxis of HSV Initiate treatment within 72 hours of symptoms
		IV 5 mg per kg^3 every eight hours	IV 5 mg per kg^3 every eight hours	Most active against HSV-1 Half as active against HSV-2
Valacyclovir	Nucleoside analogue DNA polymerase enzyme inhibitor	Oral 2000 mg twice a day	Oral 500 mg twice a day	Initiate treatment within 72 hours of symptoms Has greater bioavailability than acyclovir
Famciclovir	Guanosine nucleoside analogue	Oral 1500 mg once a day	Oral 250 mg twice a day	Initiate treatment within 72 hours of symptoms
				Has greater bioavailability than acyclovir
Pencyclovir	Acyclic guanine nucleoside analogue	Cream 1% Topical application every two hours for four days		May quicken resolution of symptoms even when applied at ulcerative phase

Anti-viral medication should be considered in cases where signs and symptoms are severe, and at an early stage [10]. It can be utilised where patients are immunocompromised. Treatment with anti-viral medication should commence within 72 hours of signs or symptoms of herpetic infection. Medications that can be used include acyclovir, valacyclovir and famciclovir. If anti-viral medication is not prescribed at an early stage, it will yield limited benefit (see Table 14.1).

Acyclovir is an acyclic guanine nucleoside analogue. Its action inhibits viral DNA synthesis, and it is highly selective for HSV-1 and HSV-2 infected cells. Its selectivity for these cells is dependent on interaction with two distinct proteins, namely, HSV thymidine kinase and DNA polymerase. Acyclovir is most active against HSV-1 and can be used in either treatment or prophylaxis of HSV. The oral bioavailability of acyclovir ranges from 10 to 30%. To avoid adverse effects, acyclovir should not be used in its topical form in immunesuppressed patients.

Another medication that is commonly used is valacyclovir. Its actions are similar to acyclovir, and it is a guanine nucleoside antiviral. Its benefit is that it has three-to-five times greater bioavailability than acyclovir. There are potential risks of neurotoxicity, and valacyclovir should not be prescribed in immune-suppressed patients. Summary of common antiviral medications against HSV is shown in Table 14.1.

Prognosis and Complications

Some patients with HSV infection may have future outbreaks (recurrences). Often it occurs at the same location signalling the latent residency of HSV within the trigeminal ganglion. To date, there is no medication available that prevents HSV from migrating to the trigeminal ganglion following a primary infection. Hence, future reaction of the disease can still occur. Typically, the more severe a primary infection is, recurrences are more likely to take place.

In patients that are immunocompromised, there is a risk or risk of a severe reoccurrence. Patients on immunosuppressive medications after transplant procedures, advanced acquired immune deficiency syndrome (AIDS) or receiving chemotherapy treatment for cancer are a few examples of patients at risk. Lesions, in these cases, may appear as enlarging ulcers. There is a risk of dissemination, leading to a generalised infection.

In general, HSV infections restricted to the oral facial–region have an excellent prognosis, despite the likelihood of future reoccurrence. Over time, repeated outbreaks have a propensity to be milder, as the body is able to produce antibodies against HSV. However, as discussed, immunocompromised persons are at risk for developing worsening HIV related symptoms. Furthermore, HSV infections of the central nervous system may have potentially fatal outcomes. Without treatment, HSV encephalitis has a mortality rate of 70% [16].

Prevention/Patient Education

Generally, to reduce the risk of transmission, patients with HSV infections should avoid direct contact with others. Recurrent herpetic conditions are extremely contagious, especially at their vesicular stage. During the vesicular stage of the infection, care should be taken to avoid autoinoculation of other mucosal sites. It is also important to avoid direct contact of the lesion. Prevention of HSV 1 and 2 is also similar to that of preventing other sexually transmitted infections. During an outbreak, sexual activity should be avoided. Correct and consistent use of condoms during sexual activities can decrease the risk of infection.

Healthcare workers treating patients with herpes virus infections need to take universal personal protective equipment precautions including the use of masks, gloves and eye protection. Currently, there is no vaccine available to prevent HSV-1 and HSV-2 infections.

Referral to a specialist in infectious diseases is recommended when patients present with severe lesions, and are immunocompromised.

References

1 World Health Organisation (2020). Herpes simplex virus [Internet]. https://www.who.int/news-room/fact-sheets/detail/herpes-simplex-virus#hsv2

2 James, C., Harfouche, M., Welton, N.J. et al. (2020). Herpes simplex virus: global infection prevalence and incidence estimates, 2016. *Bull. World Health Organ.* 98 (5): 315.

3 Sacks, S., Griffiths, P., Corey, L. et al. (2004). HSV shedding. *Antiviral Res.* 63: S19–S26.

4 Saleh, D., Yarrarapu, S.N.S., Sharma, S. (2021). Herpes simplex type 1. StatPearls [Internet]. [cited 1 September 2021] Available from: https://www.ncbi.nlm.nih.gov/books/NBK482197

5 Gnann, J.W. and Whitley, R.J. (2017). Herpes simplex encephalitis: an update. *Curr. Infect. Dis. Rep.* 19 (3): 13.

6 Atyeo, N., Rodriguez, M.D., Papp, B., and Toth, Z. (2021). Clinical manifestations and epigenetic regulation of oral herpesvirus infections. *Viruses* 13 (4): 681.

7 Arduino, P.G. and Porter, S.R. (2008). Herpes simplex virus type 1 infection: overview on relevant clinico-pathological features. *J. Oral Pathol. Med.* 37 (2): 107–121.

8 Fatahzadeh, M. and Schwartz, R.A. (2007). Human herpes simplex virus infections: epidemiology, pathogenesis, symptomatology, diagnosis, and management. *J. Am. Acad. Dermatol.* 57 (5): 737–763.

9 Balasubramaniam, R., Kuperstein, A.S., and Stoopler, E.T. (2014). Update on oral herpes virus infections. *Dental Clinics.* 58 (2): 265–280.

10 McCullough, M. and Savage, N. (2005). Oral viral infections and the therapeutic use of antiviral agents in dentistry. *Aust. Dent. J.* 50: S31–S35.

11 Kaye, S. and Choudhary, A. (2006). Herpes simplex keratitis. *Prog. Retin. Eye Res.* 25 (4): 355–380.

12 Brown, G. (1976). Herpes zoster: correlation of age, sex, distribution, neuralgia, and associated disorders. *South. Med. J.* 69 (5): 576–578.

13 Stoopler, E.T. (2005). Oral herpetic infections (HSV 1–8). *Dent. Clin.* 49 (1): 15–29.

14 Strick, L.B. and Wald, A. (2006). Diagnostics for herpes simplex virus. *Mol. Diagn. Ther.* 10 (1): 17–28.

15 Siegel, M.A. (2002). Diagnosis and management of recurrent herpes simplex infections. *J. Am. Dent. Assoc.* 133 (9): 1245–1249.

16 Jouan, Y., Grammatico-Guillon, L., Espitalier, F. et al. (2015). Long-term outcome of severe herpes simplex encephalitis: a population-based observational study. *Crit. Care* 19 (1): 1–9.

15

Human Papillomavirus Associated Oral Lesions

S.R. Prabhu[1] and Jeff Hill[2]

[1]*University of Queensland, School of Dentistry, Brisbane, Australia*
[2]*University of Alabama, School of Dentistry, Birmingham, Alabama, USA*

Introduction

Nearly every individual is infected by human papilloma virus (HPV) at some point in their lifetime [1]. Globally, HPV infection is the most common sexually transmitted viral infection in men and women [2]. HPV is responsible for benign anogenital, oral and cutaneous warts, and oropharyngeal and anogenital cancers [3]. Cervical cancer (CC) is the third most prevalent cancer in women [4]. More than 200 types of HPV have been recognised on the basis of DNA sequence. HPVs are divided into low-risk (LR) and high-risk (HR) categories. Infection with LR HPVs causes a variety of benign wart-like lesions of the skin, genital, anal and oral mucosae. Persistent infections with HR types of HPV cause cancers of cervix (~100%), anus (~88%), vagina (~78%), penis (~51%), vulva (≥25%) and oropharynx (30–70%) [5–7].

Epidemiology of Oropharyngeal Human Papillomavirus (HPV) Infection

With an estimated 291 million human papillomavirus (HPV)-positive women worldwide in 2007, HPV infection is one of the most common viral infections in the world. The first global estimate on the prevalence of oral infection derives from a systematic review published in 2010 [8] with an estimated overall oral HPV prevalence of 4.5%, and the most frequently detected HPV type was HPV16 (1.3%). In another study in 2018, the estimated overall prevalence of oral HPV infection and infection due to HPV16 were 7.7 and 1.4%, respectively [9]. Jamieson et al. in 2020 reported a high prevalence of oral HPV infection in a large sample of Indigenous Australians, with one-third testing positive [10]. Discrepancies observed in prevalence rates between studies could be partially explained by differences in risk factors for HPV infection among study populations, such as tobacco and alcohol use and differences in sexual behaviour [11].

Microbiology and Transmission

The HPV genome is composed of a double-stranded DNA molecule. The viral DNA genome encodes eight open reading frames (ORFs) comprised of six early (E1, E2, E4, E5, E6 and E7) proteins and two late (L1 and L2) proteins. Based on their association with CC and precursor lesions, HPVs are grouped as HR and LR types. LR HPVs include types 6, 11, 42, 43 and 44. HR HPVs include types 16, 18, 31, 33, 34, 35, 39, 45, 51, 52, 56, 58, 59, 66, 68 and 70 [12–14].

Transmission of HPV occurs primarily by skin-to-skin contact. HPV infection is the most common sexually transmitted infection (STI). [14] Non-sexual transmission via fomites can also occur. Multiple pathways for HPV transmission to the oral cavity exist. These include sexual transmission, autoinfection and rarely through perinatal transmission of the neonate during its passage through an infected birth canal [14, 15]. HPV can be transmitted by contact with infected labial, scrotal or anal tissues that are not protected by a condom. Oral sex is a well-recognised mode of transmission of HPV to the oral cavity [15, 16]. Oral HPV acquisition has been reported to be more positively associated with the number of recent oral sex and open mouth kissing partners than with the number of penile–vaginal sex partners. Reports also indicate that men who have sex with men (MSM) have a high risk of developing oral HPV infection [15, 16]. An individual is at greater risk of becoming infected with HPV if he or she has had multiple sexual partners or is the partner of someone who has had multiple sexual partners. Sexual activity at an early age also places an individual at increased risk, as does a history of other sexually transmitted infections (STIs), genital warts, abnormal Pap smears, or CC or penile cancer in an individual or sexual partner [15, 16]. HPV of the head and neck region is transmitted orally and oral sex has been reported to be a contributing factor to the majority of head- and neck-associated HPV transmissions/infections [17].

Pathogenesis

Normal intact skin or mucosa is resistant to inoculation by the virus [14, 18]. Through breaks in the epithelial layers, HPVs could gain entry (Figure 15.1) and infect the basal epithelial cell layers, where the virus is maintained in the nuclei of the infected cells. HPVs can infect basal epithelial cells of the skin (cutaneous types) or mucous membranes (mucosal types). Cutaneous types of HPV target the skin of the hands and feet. Mucosal types infect the anogenital epithelium, lining of the mouth, throat or respiratory tract. HPV replication cycle begins with the entry of the virus into the cells of the stratum germinativum (basal layer) of the epithelium. HPVs do not kill infected epithelial cells [14, 18]. As the basal cells of the infected epithelium divide and progress into squamous cells, HPV is carried within them. HPV needs terminally differentiated epithelial cells, such as squamous cells for replication. In the squamous cells, the virus replicates and retains a high copy number. In these cells, the viral genes are expressed, and progeny viruses are produced. These are subsequently shed into the environment [14, 18]

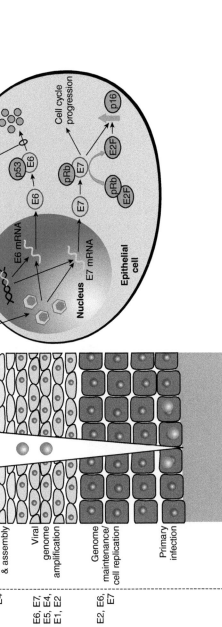

Figure 15.1 Pathogenesis of HPV infection. Human papilloma virus (HPV) infects the basal cells of the stratified squamous epithelia, which becomes exposed after wounding or micro-trauma. Virus particles are produced only in the surface of the epithelium, from where they are shed into the surroundings to infect new target cells. In the nuclei of basal cells, the viral genome remains as a low-copy plasmid. Expression of viral proteins is regulated by differentiation of the infected cells during their movement towards the epithelial surface. At an early stage of the infection, viral DNA is replicated, along with cellular DNA, during cell division at S-phase. At some point, a switch from stable replication (genome maintenance) to vegetative viral DNA replication will occur to allow the production of genomes for packaging into virions encapsulated by L1 and L2. Thousands of virus particles are produced per cell. After viral integration of high-risk HPVs, the expressions of E6 and E7 genes are permanently upregulated. HPV E6 binds and degrades p53, which leads to inhibition of apoptosis. HPV E7 protein binds and degrades the retinoblastoma tumour suppressor protein, pRB, disrupting its interaction with the transcription factor E2F. The release and activation of E2F result in expression of S-phase genes and cell-cycle progression. Upregulation of p16 is induced by HPV-mediated disruption of E7, which leads to cellular accumulation of p16. Source: Syrjänen [19] / John Wiley & Sons/CC BY-4.0

Clinical Manifestations

HPV is involved in the pathogenesis of several benign oral lesions. These include squamous cell papillomas, condyloma acuminatum, multifocal epithelial hyperplasia (Heck's Disease) and verruca vulgaris.

Oral Squamous Cell Papilloma

Oral squamous cell papilloma is caused by HPV. Viral particles closely resembling HPV have been reported in squamous papillomas [14, 17, 20, 21]. The most prevalent HPV types associated with oral squamous papillomas are HPV 6 and 11.

Oral squamous cell papilloma is a painless lesion that can occur at anywhere like tongue, lips, cheek mucosa and hard and soft palates. Most papillomas are single. The wart-like lesion is pedunculated and shows numerous papillary projections (Figure 15.2). They may be pointed, finger-like or rounded and cauliflower-like in appearance. If excessive keratinization is present, the lesion appears white. Less-keratinized lesions are often raspberry-like and pink in colour. Clinically, squamous papilloma is often indistinguishable from the common wart (verruca vulgaris). If left untreated, oral squamous cell papillomas are not known to turn into malignant lesions. Surgical excision is the treatment of choice. Once surgically removed, oral squamous papillomas usually do not recur [14, 17, 21].

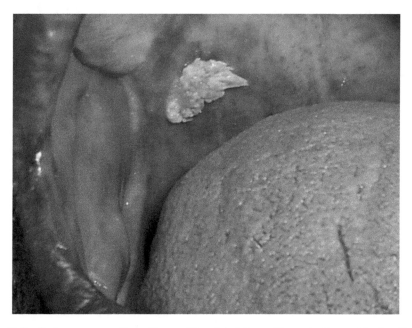

Figure 15.2   Oral squamous cell papilloma with pointed finger-like projections at the junction of hard and soft palate.

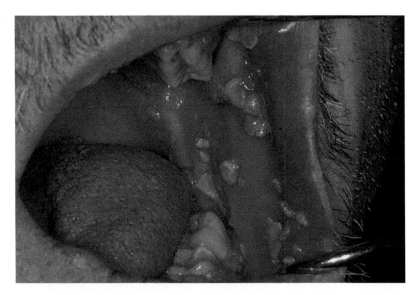

Figure 15.3 Condyloma acuminatum. This is a 44-year-old male with numerous pink/white papillary lesions, some of which are exophytic and many of which are flat and spongy. Source: Reproduced with permission from Professor Michael D. Martin of University of Washington School of Dentistry.

Oral Condyloma Acuminatum

Condyloma acuminatum, also known as the venereal/genital wart, is a STIs. This is predominantly seen on the skin and mucosal surfaces of the anogenital tract. Oral lesions occur as a result of oral sex or from autoinoculation of the virus. Common oral sites include the tongue, gingiva, soft palate and lips. Lesions are multiple and confluent, and generally larger than squamous cell papillomas [14, 17, 22, 23]. They present as broad based (sessile) pink or white cauliflower-like or mulberry-like raised lesions (Figure 15.3). Up to 50% of individuals with genital condylomas may present with oral condylomas. Oral condylomas are also frequently encountered in human immunodeficiency virus (HIV)-affected persons. HPV types, 6, 11, and 16, are associated with oral condyloma lesions. Cryotherapy, surgical excision, laser treatment and topical 5-fluorouracil are the treatment options available [14].

Multifocal Epithelial Hyperplasia

Multifocal epithelial hyperplasia, also known as Heck's disease, is predominantly a childhood disease and occasionally occurs in adults [24]. Usually, it is not sexually transmitted. Genetic pre-disposition seems to be an important factor. The aetiologic agent of multifocal epithelial hyperplasia is HPV types 13 and 32. Lesions are multiple asymptomatic, sessile and of normal mucosal colour. They are well-demarcated round to ovoid, flat lesions measuring 1–10 mm in diameter (Figure 15.4). When clustered, these lesions present a

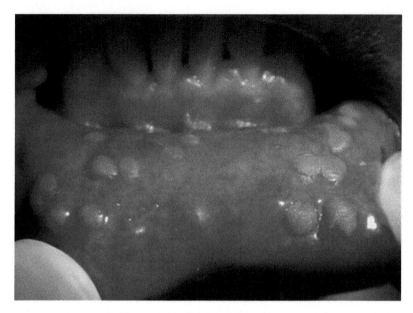

Figure 15.4 Multiple focal epithelial hyperplasia. Multiple flat and coalescent papules on the lower lip mucosa. Source: From Barroso dos Reis et al. [27] / IntechOpen, CC BY 3.

cobblestone appearance. Any part of the oral mucosa may be involved but frequent sites include lower labial mucosa, buccal mucosa, labial commissures, upper labial mucosa, tongue, gingivae, alveolar mucosa and palatal mucosa [25, 26]. Clinically, lesions resemble those of condyloma acuminatum, but lesions of multifocal epithelial hyperplasia are flatter and more numerous. Lesions heal spontaneously. Treatment is not necessary except in cases of functional or aesthetic impairment. Surgical excision, laser ablation, cryotherapy, cauterization and topical treatment with retinoic acids or interferon are available treatment options [27].

Verruca Vulgaris

Verruca vulgaris is a skin wart. Common sites of verruca vulgaris include fingers, the back of hands and feet, face, eyelids and mucocutaneous surfaces of the anogenital region. Oral warts in immunocompetent hosts are uncommon with a reported prevalence of 0.5% [14, 28]. Preferred oral sites include the labial mucosa of the lower lip and the vermilion border of lips. However, a higher prevalence of oral warts has been reported in persons with HIV and immunosuppressed persons (Figures 15.5a and b, 15.6a and b). Lesions are painless and appear as sessile, papillomatous and exophytic hyperkeratotic. Verruca vulgaris lesions are predominantly seen in children. Oral lesions generally result from autoinoculation of the virus from lesions on the fingers. When oral lesions are found, a search for skin lesions should be carried out. Verruca vulgaris is caused by HPV types 2 and 4. Oral verruca vulgaris lesions are treated with surgical removal. Recurrence is uncommon [28, 29].

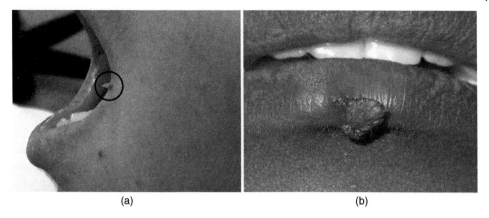

(a)   (b)

Figure 15.5   Verruca vulgaris. Exophytic lesion with hyperkeratotic surface, forming finger-like projections in the left commissure of the lip (a, circle). Lesion on the lower lip (b). Source: From Barroso dos Reis et al. [27] / IntechOpen, CC BY 3.0.

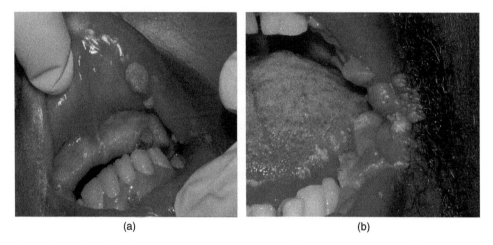

(a)   (b)

Figure 15.6   (a and b). Oral warts secondary to human papillomavirus infection in HIV patients
Source: Courtesy of David Reznik, HIVDent.Org.

HPV and Oral Potentially Malignant Disorders

Oral potentially malignant disorders (OPMDs) are a group of lesions with an increased risk of development of cancers of the oral cavity and lip. Reports indicate that the global prevalence of OPMDs is at 4.47% [30–32]. OPMDs include oral leukoplakia, oral proliferative leukoplakia, verrucous leukoplakia (VL), erythroplakia, erythroleukoplakia, oral lichen planus (OLP), oral submucous fibrosis, actinic keratosis/actinic cheilitis, palatal lesions in reverse smokers, oral lupus erythematosus, dyskeratosis congenita, oral lichenoid lesions, oral graft versus host disease and chronic hyperplastic candidosis [30–32]. Of these, three OPMDs, namely oral leukoplakia, oral proliferative verrucous leukoplakia (PVL), and OLP are known to have HPV (types 16 and 18) association. However, HPV's etiologic association has not yet been conclusively established [32]. The following sections briefly discuss the HPV association with these three oral potentially malignant disorders.

Oral Leukoplakia

Leukoplakia has been defined as 'a predominantly white plaque of questionable risk having excluded (other) known diseases or disorders that carry no increased risk for cancer' [30, 31].

Estimates of the global prevalence of oral leukoplakia range from 0.5 to 3.46%. [30–32]. Leukoplakia may be idiopathic or associated with several causes. Some known aetiologic factors of oral leukoplakia include long-term use of tobacco (smoking and smokeless) and/ or excessive alcohol consumption, chronic friction, electro-galvanic reaction caused by two dissimilar metallic restorative materials and ultraviolet radiation to the lip from chronic sun exposure. Several studies have shown that HPV types 16 and 18 are associated with oral leukoplakia lesions [17, 30, 31]. There is little evidence, however, to support a causal relationship either between HPV infection and oral leukoplakia or between HPV-infected leukoplakic keratinocytes and their carcinomatous transformation [32].

Clinically, leukoplakia is seen as a well-demarcated white/grey keratotic patch, which may appear flat, smooth, fissured, granular or nodular in appearance. The leukoplakia lesion is not removable by gentle scraping. Sometimes it may present as a red and white mixed plaque called erythroleukoplakia or speckled leukoplakia [30–32].

Leukoplakia is a potentially malignant disorder [30]. The reported prevalence of epithelial dysplasia in oral leukoplakia ranges from 5 to 25%. The presence of epithelial dysplasia is a marker of the malignant potential, and the risk of an individual leukoplakic lesion to progress to carcinoma increases with the increase of the grade (mild, moderate and severe) of the epithelial dysplasia. Globally, rates of carcinomatous transformation of oral leukoplakia range from 0.7 to 2.9% [30–33]. Oral leukoplakia needs to be distinguished from other predominantly white keratotic lesions that do not carry malignant potential. Treatment of dysplastic oral leukoplakia is done by surgical excision, laser ablation, cryosurgery or topical or systemic chemotherapy. The topical use of drugs such as β-carotene, *trans*-retinoic acid and 5-fluorouracil is useful in some cases [31–33].

Proliferative Verrucous Leukoplakia (PVL)

PVL, a distinct form of oral leukoplakia, is a potentially malignant disorder. It is a slow-growing white hyperkeratotic lesion that tends to spread and become multifocal, and it develops as a wart-like lesion over time. Gingiva and alveolar ridges are the favoured sites of PVL [30–33]. PVL has a higher rate of malignant transformation compared to other forms of oral leukoplakia [30, 31]. PVL is of unknown aetiology. An association with HPV has been suggested by some investigators. However, the causal association of the virus has not been established [33, 34].

Oral Lichen Planus (OLP)

Lichen planus (LP) is an immunologically mediated chronic mucocutaneous disorder. Often it involves only the oral mucosa with white hyperkeratotic (reticular/papular or plaque) or red erosive patterns. OLP, particularly of the erosive variant, has been considered a potentially malignant disorder with less than 2% of such lesions showing malignant transformation over a period of 10 years [30–32]. HPV DNA has been reported in up to 15.4% of cases of OLP. However, HPV's etiologic association has not been established [33, 34].

HPV and Oral and Oropharyngeal Cancers

Oral and Oropharyngeal Squamous Cell Carcinoma

Oropharyngeal squamous cell cancers (OPSCC) include cancers at the base of tongue; pharyngeal tonsils, anterior and posterior tonsillar pillars, glossotonsillar sulci; anterior surface of soft palate, uvula, and lateral and posterior pharyngeal walls. More than 90% of these cancers are squamous cell carcinomas (SCC) of the mucous membranes. Nearly 75% of oral squamous cell carcinomas (OSCC) have been attributed to smoking and alcohol consumption [35]. Despite the recent evidence of declining rates of tobacco- and alcohol-associated oral cancers, the overall incidence of oropharyngeal cancers, particularly at the base of the tongue and tonsils, is increasing. These findings reflect a possible role for risk factors other than tobacco and alcohol. In this regard, HPVs have received considerable attention in recent years. Oropharyngeal carcinomas, tonsillar cancers in particular, show the strongest association with HPV. Now there is evidence that HPV-positive OPSCC is a STI. In 2012, the International Agency of Research of Cancer (IARC) declared that there was sufficient evidence to associate a subtype of HPV 16 with oral cancers [36]. A growing body of evidence supports that approximately 20% of oral cancers and 60–80% of oropharyngeal cancers are caused by HPV [37]. According to the current literature, the risk factors of OPSCC are similar to those of CC and carcinoma in situ (CIN). The principal risk factor for CC and HPV-positive OPSCC is the sexual behaviour [38]. Evidence of HPV association with head and neck cancers through oral sex is emerging. [17] Women acquire cervical HPV through genital skin-to-skin contact, usually, but not necessarily, during sexual intercourse with an infected partner [38]. Higher risk is associated with early age at sexual exposure, multiple sexual partners and having partners who have had multiple partners [36]. The risk of HPV-positive OPSCC is primarily influenced by the lifetime number of oral sexual partners [38]. Other factors include younger age, history of genital warts and presence of other STDs. It is likely that in most HPV-related oral cancers, HPV oncogenes may also act synergistically with chemical carcinogens in alcohol, tobacco and betel quid resulting in malignant transformation of oral keratinocytes. There is evidence to suggest that HPV-related oral cancers differ from HPV-negative cancers in their clinical response and overall survival rates [39].

Oropharyngeal squamous cell carcinoma (OPSCC) refers to cancer of the tonsil, base and posterior one third of the tongue, soft palate, and posterior and lateral pharyngeal walls. Common clinical manifestations of the base of the tongue SCCs include dysphagia, odynophagia, foreign body sensation, referred otalgia, oral bleeding and a neck mass. Carcinoma may present as an indurated erythematous (Figure 15.7) or ulcerative mass. Patients may have bilateral palpable lymphadenopathy due to regional lymph node metastases. Enlarged lymph nodes may often be cystic. Approximately 70% or more of patients with advanced base-of-the-tongue cancers have ipsilateral cervical nodal metastases; 30% or fewer of such patients have bilateral, cervical lymph-node metastases [41]. Symptoms may mimic those of common upper respiratory infections. A comprehensive head and neck examination is recommended for all patients, including detailed cranial nerve examination and palpation of the neck to assess for regional metastatic lymphadenopathy. Inspection and palpation of the tongue base may be limited due to inadequate access, poor patient compliance or submucosal extent of the neoplasm. Indirect or flexible fibreoptic laryngoscopy is a useful adjunct to the physical examination. Computerized tomography (CT) scanning, magnetic resonance imaging (MRI), positron emission tomography

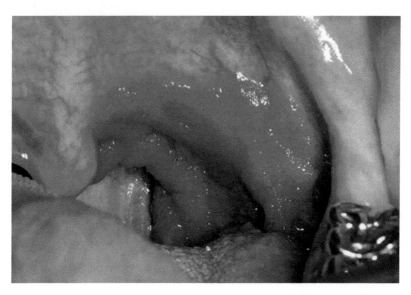

Figure 15.7 Squamous cell carcinoma. This human papillomavirus-positive tumour presented as a diffuse erythroplakia of the left soft palate and tonsillar region. Source: From Chi et al. [40] / American Cancer Society / John Wiley & Sons.

(PET)/CT scanning and ultrasonography are useful diagnostic tools [41–44]. Biopsy via endoscopic examination of the primary site with the patient under anaesthesia remains the definitive procedure to establish the diagnosis and accurately assess the primary tumour.

HPV-associated oropharyngeal SCC frequently lacks keratinization and mature squamous differentiation, unlike the traditional, keratinizing SCC associated with tobacco and alcohol use. Testing with p16 immuno-histochemistry is required for all newly diagnosed base of tongue SCCs, with p16 overexpression being strongly associated with HR HPV. Additional HPV testing such as in situ hybridization or polymerase chain reaction (PCR) assay can be utilised to clarify HPV status [41–44].

Four types of standard treatment are used for oropharyngeal SCCs: surgery, radiation therapy, chemotherapy and targeted therapy. Immunotherapy is being tested in clinical trials. Patients with HPV-positive OPSCC seem to have significantly better response to chemotherapy and radiotherapy as compared with HPV-negative OPSCCs. These patients also seem to have a lower risk of a second primary cancer. The overall five-year survival rate in patients with oropharyngeal cancer is about 60%. Prognosis of OPSCC varies with the cause. Patients who are HPV-positive have a five-year survival of >75% (and a three-year survival of almost 90%), whereas HPV-negative patients have a five-year survival of <50% [41–44].

Oral Verrucous Carcinoma

Oral verrucous carcinoma (OVC), also known as Ackerman's tumour, is a variant of OSCC. OVC presents as an exophytic, soft, fungating, painless, slow growing and locally aggressive tumour. A strong aetiological association with tobacco and alcohol has been reported for the development of OVC. HPV DNA types 6, 11, 16 and 18 have also been shown to be associated with OVC by some investigators [45]. The role of HPV in the causation of OVC is controversial [46]. OVC responds well to surgical management, but recurrences are common.

Prevention of HPV-Positive Oral Lesions

Early Detection of HPV-Positive Oral Lesions

From the above discussion, it is evident that HPV is present in the normal oral mucosa and is associated with potentially malignant disorders such as oral leukoplakia and LP and in OSCC. This points to the strong possibility that some link between HPV infection and oral potentially malignant and cancerous lesions does exist. It is important that such suspicious lesions be detected by combining HPV type with exfoliative cytology. As chemical carcinogens in tobacco and alcohol appear to enhance HPV-transforming activity, patients with positive oral cytology should be strongly advised to reduce or discontinue their use. Patient education on risk factors for oral cancer and OPMDs should include oral HPV transmission related to sexual practices.

HPV Vaccines

HPV vaccination works extremely well as a preventive measure for CC. Centre for Disease Control and Prevention (CDC) recommends HPV vaccination for 11- to 12-year-olds and for everyone through age 26 years, if not vaccinated already. Three HPV vaccines – 9-valent HPV vaccine (Gardasil 9, 9vHPV), quadrivalent HPV vaccine (Gardasil, 4vHPV) and bivalent HPV vaccine (Cervarix, 2vHPV) – have been licensed by the U.S. Food and Drug Administration (FDA). All three HPV vaccines protect against HPV types 16 and 18 that cause most HPV cancers. Since late 2016, only Gardasil-9 (9vHPV) has been distributed in the United States. This vaccine protects against nine HPV types (6, 11, 16, 18, 31, 33, 45, 52 and 58) (see https://www.cdc.gov/vaccines/vpd/hpv/public/index.html) [47, 48]. Vaccines are recommended for females aged 9–25, who have not been exposed to HPV. It is possible that currently available HPV vaccines designed to prevent CCs and genital warts will also contribute to the reduction in the incidence of HPV-related oropharyngeal cancers. A recent study suggests that HPV vaccines can protect against oral vaccine-type HPV infection including high-risk HPV16 infection, thus reducing the incidence of HPV-related oro-pharyngeal cancer (OPC). Vaccination against HPV, especially in males, who are predominantly affected by HPV-related OPSCC, could result in the prevention of this disease [49]. Therapeutic HPV vaccines, which are being developed for CC, may also be of benefit in the management of HPV-related oral cancer.

References

1 Chesson, H.W., Dunne, E.F., Hariri, S., and Markowitz, L.E. (2014). The estimated lifetime probability of acquiring human papillomavirus in the United States. *Sex. Transm. Dis.* 41: 660–664. https://doi.org/10.1097/OLQ.0000000000000193.

2 World Health Organization. (2019). Human papillomavirus (HPV) and cervical cancer [fact sheet]. Available from: https://www.who.int/en/news-room/fact-sheets/detail/human-papillomavirus-(hpv)-and-cervical-cancer.

3 De Martel, C., Plummer, M., Vignat, J., and Franceschi, S. (2017). Worldwide burden of cancer attributable to HPV by site, country, and HPV type. *Int. J. Cancer* 141: 664–670. https://doi.org/10.1002/ijc.30716.

4 Bruni, L., Albero, G., Serrano, B. et al. (2019). ICO/IARC information centre on HPV and cancer (HPV Information Centre). Human Papillomavirus and Related Diseases in the World. Summary Report. https://www.hpvcentre.net/statistics/reports/XWX.pdf

5 Plummer, M., de Martel, C., Vignat, J. et al. (2016). Global burden of cancers attributable to infections in 2012: a synthetic analysis. *Lancet Glob. Health* 4: e609–e616. https://doi .org/10.1016/s2214-109x(16)30143-7.

6 Ndiaye, M., Mena, L., Alemany, M. et al. (2014). HPV DNA, E6/E7 mRNA, and p16INK4a detection in head and neck cancers: a systematic review and meta-analysis. *Lancet Oncol.* 15: 1319–1331. https://doi.org/10.1016/s1470-2045(14)70471-1.

7 Mehanna, H.T., Beech, T., Nicholson, I. et al. (2013). Prevalence of human papillomavirus in oropharyngeal and nonoropharyngeal head and neck cancer—systematic review and meta-analysis of trends by time and region. *Head Neck* 35: 747–755. https://doi.org/ 10.1002/hed.22015.

8 Kreimer, A.R., Bhatia, R.K., Messeguer, A.L. et al. (2010). Oral human papillomavirus in healthy individuals: a systematic review of the literature. *Sex. Transm. Dis.* 37: 386–391.

9 Tam, S., Fu, S., Xu, L. et al. (2018). The epidemiology of oral human papillomavirus infection in healthy populations: a systematic review and meta-analysis. *Oral Oncol.* 2018 (82): 91–99.

10 Jamieson, L.M., Antonsson, A., Garvey, G. et al. (2020, 2020). Prevalence of Oral human papillomavirus infection among Australian indigenous adults. *JAMA Netw. Open* 3 (6): e204951. https://doi.org/10.1001/jamanetworkopen.2020.4951. PMID: 32511719; PMCID: PMC7280951.

11 Mena, M., Taberna, M., Monfil, L. et al. (2019). Might Oral human papillomavirus (HPV) infection in healthy individuals explain differences in HPV-attributable fractions in oropharyngeal Cancer? A systematic review and Meta-analysis. *J Infect Dis* 219 (10): 1574–1585. https://doi.org/10.1093/infdis/jiy715.

12 World Health Organization (2007). International Agency for Researchon Cancer (IARC). Human papillomaviruses. *IARC MonogrEval Carcinog Risk Hum.* 90: 47–79.

13 de Villeirs, E.M. and Gunst, K. (2009). Characterisation of seven novel human papillomavirus types isolated from cutaneous tissue, but also present in mucosal lesions. *J. Gen. Virol.* 90: 1994–2004.

14 Prabhu, S.R. and Wilson, D.F. (2013). Human papillomavirus and oral disease – emerging evidence: a review. *Aust. Dent. J.* 58 (1): 2–10; quiz 125. https://doi.org/10.1111/adj.12020. Epub 2013 Jan 31. PMID: 23441786.

15 Edwards, A. and Carne, C. (1998). Oral sex and the transmission of viral STIs. *Sex. Transm. Infect.* 74: 6–10.

16 Centers for Disease Control and Prevention (CDC) (2021). *Sexually Transmitted Disease Risk and Oral Sex.* Fact Sheet https://www.cdc.gov/std/healthcomm/stdfact-stdriskandoralsex.htm.

17 Tumban, E. (2019). A current update on human papillomavirus-associated head and neck cancers. *Viruses* 11 (10): 922. https://doi.org/10.3390/v11100922. PMID: 31600915; PMCID: PMC6833051.

18 World Health Organization International. Agency for Research on Cancer (IARC) (2007). Human Papillomaviruses. *IARC Monogr Eval Carcinog Risk Hum.* 90: 130–179.

19 Syrjänen, S. (2018). Oral manifestations of human papillomavirus infections. *Eur. J. Oral Sci.* 126 (Suppl 1): 49–66. http://doi.org/10.1111/eos.12538. PMID: 30178562; PMCID: PMC6174935. http://creativecommons.org/licenses/by/4.0/Licence.

20 Betz, S.J. (2019). HPV-related papillary lesions of the oral mucosa: a review. *Head Neck Pathol.* 13 (1): 80–90. https://doi.org/10.1007/s12105-019-01003-7. Epub 2019 Jan 29. PMID: 30693456; PMCID: PMC6405797.

21 Eversole, L.R. and Laipis, P.J. (1998). Oral squamous papillomas: detection of HPV DNA by in situ hybridization. *Oral Surg. Oral Med. Oral Pathol.* 65: 545–550.

22 Choukas, N.C. and Toto, P.D. (1965). Condyloma accuminatum of the oral cavity. *Oral Surg. Oral Med. Oral Pathol.* 54: 480–485.

23 Eversole, L.R., Laipis, P.J., Merrell, P., and Choi, E. (1998). Demonstration of human papillomavirus DNA in oral condyloma acuminatum. *J. Oral Pathol.* 16: 266–272.

24 Archard, H., Heck, J.W., and Stanley, H.R. (1965). Focal epithelial hyperplasia: an unusual oral mucosal lesion found in Indian children. *Oral Surg.* 20: 201–212.

25 Santos, C., Marta de Castro, M., Benevdes dos Santos, P. et al. (2006). Oral focal epithelial hyperplasia: report of five cases. *Braz. Dent. J.* 17 (79–82): 47.

26 Hashemipour, M.A. and Shoryabi, A. (2010). Extensive focal epithelial hyperplasia. *Arch. Arab. Med.* 13: 48–52.

27 dos Reis, H.L.B., de Oliveira, S.P., Camisasca, D.R. et al. (2014). Oral HPV related diseases: a review and an update. In: *Trends in Infectious Diseases* (ed. S.K. Saxena). IntechOpen, http://doi.org/10.5772/57574. https://www.intechopen.com/chapters/46324#F1.

28 Eversole, L.R. (2000). Papillary lesions of the oral cavity: relationship to human papillomaviruses. *J. Calif. Dent. Assoc.* 28: 922–927.

29 Scully, C., Prime, S., and Maitland, N. (1985). Papillomaviruses: their role in oral disease. *Oral Surg. Oral Med. Oral Pathol.* 60: 166–174.

30 Warnakulasuriya, S. (2020). Oral potentially malignant disorders: a comprehensive review on clinical aspects and management. *Oral Oncology* 102: 104550. https://doi.org/10.1016/j.oraloncology.2019.104550.

31 Warnakulasuriya, S., Johnson, N.W., and van der Waal, I. (2007). Nomenclature and classification of potentially malignant disorders of the oral mucosa. *J. Oral Pathol. Med.* 36: 575–580.58.

32 Locca, O., Sollecito, T.P., Alawi, F. et al. (2020). Potentially malignant disorders of the oral cavity and oral dysplasia: a systematic review and meta-analysis of malignant transformation rate by subtype. *Head Neck* 42: 539–555.

33 Kashima, H.K., Kutcher, M., Kessis, T. et al. (1990). Human papillomavirus in squamous cell carcinoma, leukoplakia, lichen planus, and clinically normal epithelium of the oral cavity. *Ann. Otol. Rhinol. Laryngol.* 99: 55–61.

34 Campisi, G., Giovannelli, L., Ammatuna, P. et al. (2004). Proliferative verrucous vs conventional leukoplakia: no significantly increased risk of HPV infection. *Oral Oncol.* 40: 835–840.

35 Warnakulasuriya, S. (2009). Global epidemiology of oral and oropharyngeal cancer. *Oral Oncol.* 45: 309–316.

36 IARC Working Group on the Evaluation of Carcinogenic Risks to Humans (2012). *ARC Monographs on The Evaluation of Carcinogenic Risks to Humans: IARC Monographs, 100B. A Review of Human Carcinogens. B. Biological agents*, 278–280. Lyon: International Agency for Research on Cancer.

37 Syrjänen, S., Lodi, G., Bültzingslöwen, I. et al. (2011). Human papillomaviruses in oral carcinoma and oral potentially malignant disorders: a systematic review. *Oral Dis. Suppl.* 1: 58–72. http://doi.org/10.1111/j.1601-0825.2011.01792.x.

38 Berman, T.A. and Schiller, J.T. (2017). Human papillomavirus in cervical cancer and oropharyngeal cancer: one cause, two diseases. *Cancer* 2017 123: 2219–2229.

39 Fakhry, C., Westra, W.H., Li, S. et al. (2008). Improved survival of patients with human papillomavirus-positive head and neck squamous cell carcinoma in a prospective clinical trial. *J. Natl. Cancer Inst.* 100: 261–269.

40 Chi, A.C., Day, T.A., and Neville, B.W. (2015). Oral cavity and oropharyngeal squamous cell carcinoma—an update. *CA: A Cancer Journal for Clinicians* 65 (5): 401–421.

41 Choi, W.H., Hu, K.S., Culliney, B. et al. (2009). Cancer of the oropharynx. In: *Head and Neck Cancer: A Multidisciplinary Approach*, 3e (ed. L.B. Harrison, R.B. Sessions and W.K. Hong), 285–335. William & Wilkins: Lippincott.

42 Tahari, A.K., Alluri, K.C., Quon, H. et al. (2014). FDG PET/CT imaging of oropharyngeal squamous cell carcinoma: characteristics of human papillomavirus-positive and -negative tumors. *Clin. Nucl. Med.* 39 (3): 225–231.

43 Tabor, M.P., Braakhuis, B.J., van der Wal, J.E. et al. (2003). Comparative molecular and histological grading of epithelial dysplasia of the oral cavity and the oropharynx. *J. Pathol.* 199 (3): 354–360.

44 PDQ® Adult Treatment Editorial Board. PDQ Oropharyngeal Cancer Treatment (Adult). Bethesda, MD: National Cancer Institute. Available at: https://www.cancer.gov/types/head-and-neck/hp/adult/oropharyngeal-treatment-pdq.

45 Cuesta, K.H., Palazzo, J.P., and Mittal, K.R. (1998). Detection of human papillomavirus in verrucous carcinoma from HIV-seropositive patients. *J. Cutan. Pathol.* 25: 165–170.

46 del Pino, M., Bleeker, M., Quint, W. et al. (2012). Comprehensive analysis of human papillomavirus prevalence and the potential role of low-risk types in verrucous carcinoma. *Mod. Pathol.* 25: 1354–1363. https://doi.org/10.1038/modpathol.2012.91.

47 Harper, D.M., Franco, E.L., and Wheeler, C.M. (2006). Sustained efficacy up to 4.5 years of a bivalent L1 virus-like particle vaccine against human papilloma virus types 16 and 18: follow-up from a randomised control trial. *Lancet* 367: 1247–1255.

48 Mannarini, L., Kratochvil, V., Calabrese, L. et al. (2009). Human papillomavirus (HPV) in head and neck region: review of literature. *Acta Otorhinolaryngol. Ital.* 29: 119–126.

49 Tsentemeidou, A., Fyrmpas, G., Stavrakas, M. et al. (2021). Human papillomavirus vaccine to end oropharyngeal Cancer. A systematic review and meta-analysis. *Sex. Transm. Dis.* 48 (9): 700–707. https://doi.org/10.1097/OLQ.0000000000001405.

16

Oropharyngeal Manifestations of Chlamydia

Nicholas van Wagoner[1] and S.R. Prabhu[2]

[1]Department of Infectious Diseases, University of Alabama at Birmingham, Heersink School of Medicine, Birmingham, AL, USA
[2]University of Queensland, School of Dentistry, Brisbane, Australia

Introduction

Chlamydia is a common sexually transmitted infection (STI) caused by infection with *Chlamydia trachomatis*. The species *C. trachomatis* exclusively infects humans. Cervicitis in females and urethritis in males are commonly caused by *C. trachomatis*. Oropharyngeal infection has also been reported both in men and women [1, 2].

Epidemiology

C. trachomatis is the most reported bacterial sexually transmitted infection (STI) in the world, with high occurrence among men who have sex with men (MSM) [1, 2]. There are relatively few epidemiological studies investigating the extragenital transmission of chlamydia by sexual practices other than anal and oral sex in MSM. The prevalence of pharyngeal *C. trachomatis* in MSM ranges from 0.5 to 3.6% (median: 1.7%) [2]. An Australian study found that men who often engaged in receptive oral–penile sex with ejaculation were 5.3 times more likely to have oropharyngeal chlamydia compared to men who never had receptive penile–oral sex with ejaculation with their casual partners in the last six months [3]. Another study found that among female sex workers, the prevalence of oropharyngeal chlamydia was similar to the prevalence at genital sites and is often independent of genital infection [4].

Aetiology/Risk Factors/Transmission

C. trachomatis is an obligate intracellular bacterium with a cell wall and ribosomes similar to those of Gram-negative organisms. Risk factors associated with acquisition of chlamydial

Sexually Transmissible Oral Diseases, First Edition.
Edited by S.R. Prabhu, Nicholas van Wagoner, Jeff Hill and Shailendra Sawleshwarkar.

infection include new or multiple sex partners, a history of STIs, presence of another STI, and lack of barrier contraception. Giving oral sex to a partner with an infected penis can also result in getting chlamydia in the throat. Sexually acquired *C. trachomatis* is highly transmissible. Transmission of *C. trachomatis* can also occur from mother to infant via the genital tract during birth [1–5].

Clinical Manifestations

In patients, who develop symptomatic infection, the incubation period for *C. trachomatis* infection is estimated to be 7–21 days. *C. trachomatis* can cause anogenital infections, lymphogranuloma venereum (LGV), conjunctivitis and oropharyngeal infection in adults, and conjunctivitis and pneumonia in neonates.

In women, the bacteria initially infect the cervix, where the infection may cause signs and symptoms of cervicitis (e.g. mucopurulent endocervical discharge and easily induced endocervical bleeding), and sometimes the urethra, which may result in signs and symptoms of urethritis (e.g. pyuria, dysuria and urinary frequency). Infection can spread from the cervix to the upper reproductive tract (i.e. uterus and fallopian tubes), causing pelvic inflammatory disease (PID), which may be asymptomatic ('subclinical PID') or acute, with typical symptoms of abdominal and/or pelvic pain, along with signs of cervical motion tenderness and uterine or adnexal tenderness on examination [6–9].

Men who are symptomatic typically have urethritis, with a mucoid or watery urethral discharge and dysuria. A minority of infected men develop epididymitis (with or without symptomatic urethritis), presenting with unilateral testicular pain, tenderness and swelling [6–9].

Chlamydia can infect the rectum in men and women, either directly (through receptive anal sex), or possibly via spread from the cervix and vagina in a woman with cervical chlamydial infection. While these infections are often asymptomatic, they can cause symptoms of proctitis (e.g. rectal pain, discharge and/or bleeding) [6–9].

Oropharyngeal Infection

Oropharyngeal infection with *C. trachomatis* most frequently is asymptomatic in both men and women. It can also present as acute tonsillitis, acute pharyngitis or abnormal pharyngeal sensation syndrome [1, 6, 9, 10]. When clinical signs and symptoms are described, the presentation can range from minimally symptomatic disease (i.e. dry or pruritic throat) to exudative tonsillopharyngitis. Chlamydial tonsillopharyngitis is marked by generalised pharyngeal and tonsillar hyperaemia with possible addition of swollen anterior pillars and uvula, as well as diffuse purulent exudate on the tonsils [1, 6, 9].

Diagnosis

Rectal and oropharyngeal *C. trachomatis* infection among persons engaging in receptive anal or oral intercourse can be diagnosed by testing at the anatomic exposure site. There are a number of diagnostic tests for chlamydia, including nucleic acid amplification tests (NAATs), cell culture and serology. NAATs are the most sensitive tests and can be performed on easily obtainable specimens such as vaginal swabs (either clinician- or patient-collected) or urine. Vaginal swabs, either patient- or clinician-collected, are the optimal specimen to screen for genital chlamydia using NAATs in women; urine is the specimen of choice for men. NAATs have demonstrated improved sensitivity and specificity compared with culture for the detection of *C. trachomatis* at rectal and oropharyngeal sites [7, 8].

Treatment

Chlamydia can be easily cured with antibiotics. The preferred treatment for chlamydia is *doxycycline* 100 mg for 7days. Azithromycin is an alternative treatment option. Persons with chlamydia should abstain from sexual activity until completion of completion of the seven day course of antibiotics or for seven days after single dose antibiotic to prevent spreading the infection [8–10].

Adults with Oropharyngeal Chlamydial Infections

Since Oropharyngeal *C. trachomatis* can be transmitted to genital sites of sex partners, detection of *C. trachomatis* from an oropharyngeal sample warrants treatment as described above [8–10].

Prevention/Patient Education

Latex male condoms, when used consistently and correctly, can reduce the risk of getting or giving chlamydia. The surest way to avoid chlamydia is to abstain from vaginal, anal and oral sex, or have a sex partner that has been tested for chlamydia, is known to be uninfected and has no other sex partners [6, 10].

References

1 Spach, D.H. and Jordan, S. (2021). Chlamydia: Core concepts. National STD Curriculum. University of Washington, USA. https://www.std.uw.edu/go/comprehensive-study/chlamydia/core-concept/all

2 Evers, Y.J., Dukers-Muijrers, N.H.T.M., van Liere, G.A.F.S. et al. (2021). Pharyngeal *Chlamydia trachomatis* in men who have sex with men (MSM) in The Netherlands: a large retrospective cohort study. *Clin. Infect. Dis.* 2021: ciab685. https://doi.org/10.1093/cid/ciab685.

3 Templeton, D.J., Jin, F., Imrie, J. et al. (2008). Prevalence, incidence and risk factors for pharyngeal chlamydia in the community-based health in men (HIM) cohort of homosexual men in Sydney, Australia. *Sex. Transm. Infect.* 84 (5): 361–363.

4 Chow, E.P., Williamson, D.A., Fortune, R. et al. (2019). Prevalence of genital and oropharyngeal chlamydia and gonorrhoea among female sex workers in Melbourne, Australia, 2015–2017: need for oropharyngeal testing. *Sex. Transm. Infect.* 95 (6): 398–401. https://doi.org/10.1136/sextrans-2018-053957. Epub 2019 May 21. PMID: 31113904.

5 Newman, L., Rowley, J., Vander Hoorn, S. et al. (2015). Global estimates of the prevalence and incidence of four curable sexually transmitted infections in 2012 based on systematic review and global reporting. *PLoS One* 10: e0143304.

6 Chlymidia-Fact sheet (Detailed) CDC (2021). Division of STD Prevention, National Center for HIV, Viral Hepatitis, STD, and TB Prevention, Centers for Disease Control and Prevention

7 Schachter, J., Chernesky, M.A., Willis, D.E. et al. (2005). Vaginal swabs are the specimens of choice when screening for *Chlamydia trachomatis* and *Neisseria gonorrhoeae*: results from a multicenter evaluation of the APTIMA assays for both infections. *Sex. Transm. Dis.* 32: 725–728.

8 Workowski, K.A., Bachmann, L.H., Chang, P.A. et al. (2021). Sexually transmitted infections treatment guidelines, 2021. *MMWR Recomm. Rep.* 70 (4): 1–187.

9 Chan, P.A., Robinette, A., Montgomery, M. et al. (2016). Extragenital Infections Caused by *Chlamydia trachomatis* and *Neisseria gonorrhoeae*: A Review of the Literature. *Infect. Dis. Obstet. Gynecol.* 2016: 5758387, 17 pages. https://doi.org/10.1155/2016/5758387.

10 Chlamydial infection among adolescents and adults. (2021). STI Treatment Guidelines. CDC.

17

Oropharyngeal Manifestations of Infectious Mononucleosis

Sue-Ching Yeoh

The Chris O'Brien Life house, Camperdown NSW, Australia

Introduction

Infectious mononucleosis (IM) ('mono' or 'glandular fever') is a common infection caused by Epstein–Barr virus (EBV), a member of the Human Herpes Virus (HHV) family. This is not a classic sexually transmitted infection, but it is included in this chapter because it is transmitted through intimate inter-personal contact and is usually transmitted by contaminated saliva. Kissing is the major route of transmission of primary EBV infection among adolescents and young adults.

IM was recognised in the 1880s by a Russian paediatrician, Nil Filatov, as a syndrome which he called 'idiopathic adenitis' [1]. The condition was then noted by German physicians in 1889 and termed 'Drüsenfieber' (glandular fever). IM was subsequently formally described by Sprunt and Evans in the Bulletin of the Johns Hopkins Hospital in 1920 in a paper entitled 'Mononuclear leukocytosis in reaction to acute infection (IM)' because the causative organism, EBV, had yet to be described [2].

Features of classic IM consist of fever, cervical lymphadenopathy and pharyngitis, accompanied by atypical large peripheral blood lymphocytes. The infection is usually transmitted by infected saliva, and individuals infected prior to adolescence rarely develop the classic symptoms.

Epidemiology

Epidemiological studies have demonstrated two peaks of infection: the first in preschool aged children (one to six years of age), and the second in adolescents and young adults [3]. Infection with EBV is common worldwide. Positive antibodies have been noted in 90% of adults before the age of 30. There is a lower prevalence of EBV antibodies in preadolescent children ranging from 20 to 80%, with the variation linked

Sexually Transmissible Oral Diseases, First Edition.
Edited by S.R. Prabhu, Nicholas van Wagoner, Jeff Hill and Shailendra Sawleshwarkar.
© 2023 John Wiley & Sons Ltd. Published 2023 by John Wiley & Sons Ltd.

to factors such as geographic region, race/ethnicity, socioeconomic status, crowding or sharing a bedroom, maternal education and day-care attendance [4]. In the United States, antibody prevalence in children of 6–19 years old is significantly higher in African Americans and Mexican Americans than in Caucasians. This disparity is greatest in the six to eight year old group but diminishes during the teenage years [4]. There is no obvious gender predilection.

Aetiopathogenesis

EBV is mostly transmitted by repeated contact with infected oropharyngeal secretions. Adults seem to be most contagious 30–50 days following infection, whereas in children, the most contagious period is 10–14 days following infection [5].

The virus enters the body via epithelial cells of the oropharynx, and can be detected in saliva, blood and lymphatics. Viral invasion of B lymphocytes is via the CD21 receptors, and viral antigen is detectable within the lymphocyte nucleus within 18–24 hours. The signs and symptoms of infection are attributable to the process of viral replication and the host immune response. The infection spreads throughout the reticuloendothelial system by the infected B lymphocytes, and both humoral and cellular immune responses are activated. B-lymphocyte proliferation into plasma cells and immortalisation into memory B lymphocytes occurs without T-helper cell involvement.

Not all of the plasma cells produce antibodies to EBV antigens. Some produce antibodies that react with cattle and sheep erythrocytes (heterophile response), and this feature is used for serological screening for IM (Monospot test). Other plasma cells produce antibodies that react with EBV antigens, which may be used to confirm a diagnosis of IM. Natural killer cells and CD8 cytotoxic T cells control proliferating B lymphocytes infected with EBV.

During the acute phase of infection, as many as 20% of the circulating B lymphocytes will produce EBV antigens, whereas only 1% will produce them during recovery. The virus usually is not found freely circulating but is commonly present as immune complexes, thought to be responsible for the arthralgias and urticarial rashes that occur during the acute phase of the disease. Viral-directed cytolysis eliminates the B lymphocytes that produce complete virions. Cytotoxic T cells target and control the proliferation of the infected B lymphocytes that do not produce complete virions. The lymphocytosis often noted in IM patients is caused by an increase in the number of circulating activated T and B lymphocytes. $CD8^+$ T cells increase in numbers in circulating blood. Their activation leads to elimination of virally infected B lymphocytes. The activated T cells are also known as Downey cells, reactive lymphocytes or atypical lymphocytes due to their atypical presence in peripheral blood. EBV is never completely cleared from the body, even after clinical recovery. The virus can be detected in oropharyngeal washings up to 18 months after the patient has fully recovered [6].

Microbiology

EBV is classified in the family Herpesviridiae, subfamily Gamaherpesvirinae, genus *Lymphocryptovirus* and species HHV 4. It is a double-stranded DNA virus. Once the virus has entered the body, it reproduces and via a process called 'shedding' becomes detectable in saliva. EBV transmission generally occurs via contact with oropharyngeal secretions containing the virus. Kissing is the main route of transmission of primary EBV infection amongst adolescents and young adults. Transmission can also occur through blood and blood-derivative transfusions as well as by organ or tissue transplantation. Breast milk of an infected mother may also contain the virus, but this is thought to be an uncommon route of vertical transmission. EBV is also present in genital tract secretions.

The incubation period of IM is approximately six weeks. The primary EBV infection can result in the classic mucocutaneous features of IM; or may results in an acute EBV-associated syndrome, such as haemophagocytic syndrome or Gianotti–Crosti syndrome. Two types of chronic active EBV infection have been noted. These are chronic EBV with persistent IM-like illness, having a good prognosis; and severe chronic EBV infections that having severe, manifestations and a significantly poorer prognosis.

Like all herpesviruses, EBV establishes persistent life-long infection without causing disease in most people. In some cases, latent EBV infection may result in various conditions, such as hydroa vacciniforme, oral hairy leukoplakia, and various lymphoproliferative disorders. Latent infection has also been linked to nasopharyngeal carcinoma, Burkitt lymphoma, Hodgkin lymphoma, and Kikuchi histocytic necrotizing lymphadenitis.

Clinical Features

Most affected children are asymptomatic; however, in young adults, symptoms like fever, lymphadenopathy, pharyngitis and tonsillitis are noted (Figure 17.1a,b). Prodromal

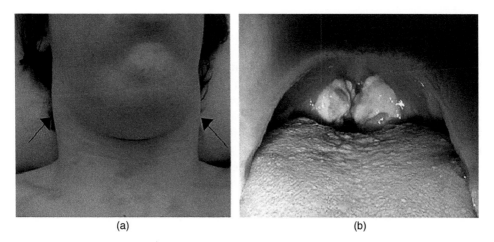

(a)   (b)

Figure 17.1   (a). Swollen cervical lymph nodes (arrows) and (b) exudative pharyngitis in a person with infectious mononucleosis. Source: James Heilman/Wikipedia Commons/CC BY-SA 3.0.

symptoms of malaise and fatigue precede the development of fever by two weeks. The classic symptoms then last for 2–14 days in most cases [5]. Patients may also develop nausea and abdominal pain due to hepatosplenomegaly. Arthralgia may also be a feature of IM.

Oropharyngeal lesions of IM characteristically consist of pharyngitis and petechial haemorrhages of the soft palate and oropharynx, usually in young adults with concomitant fever and cervical lymphadenopathy. Necrotising ulcerative gingivitis may also develop. In the majority of cases, IM lymphadenopathy is present and the cervical lymph nodes are most commonly involved, although generalised lymphadenopathy may occur. Salivary gland enlargement may also be observed.

Systemic symptoms associated with IM are often helpful in distinguishing the oral manifestations of the condition from clinically similar lesions, such as oral and pharyngeal petechiae secondary to fellatio and violent coughing or sneezing. Oral complications are rare. Cranial nerve deficit following an acute episode of IM has been reported, as well as cervical abscess, parotid mass with facial nerve palsy and lingual tonsillitis.

Once symptoms from the primary infection have resolved, the EBV will remain dormant in the body and can reactivate periodically. This does not usually trigger symptoms; however, it should be noted that the individual is potentially infectious during this time. When children are affected by the virus, they usually have either very mild symptoms or no obvious illness.

Differential Diagnosis

Several non-EBV infections may present with mononucleosis-like features. These include cytomegalovirus (CMV), human immunodeficiency virus (HIV), toxoplasma, HHV type 6 (HHV-6), streptococcal pharyngitis, hepatitis B and HHV-7. These should be considered in the differential diagnosis, in cases where the heterophile test is negative.

Diagnosis/Investigations

The diagnosis of IM is commonly based on clinical findings. IM should be suspected in patients of 10–30 years of age, who present with sore throat and significant fatigue, palatal petechiae, posterior cervical or auricular adenopathy, marked axillary adenopathy or inguinal adenopathy [6]. Lymphocytosis and the presence of atypical lymphocytes in peripheral blood smears are highly suggestive of IM (Figure 17.2) in the presence of other associated clinical signs and symptoms.

Rapid serologic tests, for example, heterophile antibody (monospot test or Paul–Bunnell test) are available. In this test, the heterophile antibody against EBV cross-reacts and agglutinates with sheep red blood cells. EBV-specific antibody is confirmatory of IM [7]. In some patients, abnormal hepatic function may be observed.

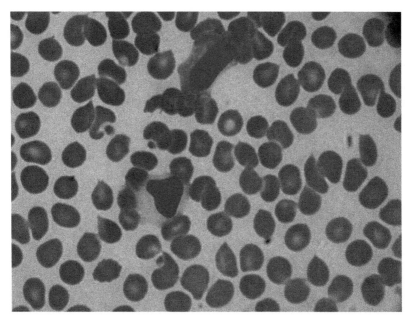

Figure 17.2 Infectious mononucleosis. Peripheral smear, high power showing reactive lymphocytes with large irregular nuclei. Source: James Heilman/Wikipedia Commons/CC BY 2.0.

Management/Treatment Considerations (of Oral Lesions)

The classic oropharyngeal lesions of IM usually require no treatment and resolve spontaneously within four to six weeks [8], with patients only requiring supportive treatment for clinical symptoms. Nonsteroidal anti-inflammatory drugs are used for fever reduction and bed rest is advised.

IM is, in most cases, self-limiting; however, the incidence and prevalence of chronic EBV infection continue to be a source of great debate [9]. Acyclovir has been proposed for use in the early stages of the disease but is still a matter of contention [10]. In some cases, corticosteroids may be prescribed to manage the inflammatory complications of the infection, such as airway obstruction, but this practice remains controversial, particularly, as it may impair clearance of the virus [11].

Patients who are prescribed ampicillin or amoxicillin may develop a pink maculopapular cutaneous rash.

Prognosis

Prognosis of patients with IM is generally good. Recovery can be monitored with serial full blood counts which should demonstrate normalisation of the lymphocytosis over times.

Positive heterophile test results may be noted for up to one year after infection [5]. Serial specific EBV antibody testing is usually not necessary in patients with acute infection. Increased immunoglobulin G (IgG), viral capsid antigen (VCA) and EBV nuclear antigen (EBNA) levels persist for life, with varying titres. IgG titres have no clear relationship to disease activity or to how the patient feels. Fatigue may take some time to resolve, and some patients may develop a state of chronic fatigue that is induced, but not caused by, EBV IM.

Complications

During the acute phase of infection, extreme oropharyngeal inflammation may result in airway obstruction. Encephalitis, myocarditis, haemolytic anaemia and thrombocytopenia occur in 1% of patients. Splenic rupture has been noted in <1% of patients, and patients should be advised not to participate in contact sports for three weeks after full clinical recovery [12].

Some patients develop chronic active EBV and may exhibit the classic signs and symptoms of IM for a prolonged period of time. These patients also demonstrate high levels of EBV DNA in the blood. Rarely, patients may develop lymphoma. EBV infection has also been associated with several other diseases such as Burkitt's lymphoma, Hodgkin's lymphoma, nasopharyngeal carcinoma and gastric carcinoma. The association between previous IM and the development of these neoplasms is still unclear [13].

Referral/Prevention/Patient Education

Spread of EBV can be prevented through careful hand hygiene especially after sneezing and coughing, and before touching other people. Patients with active IM should avoid exposing other people to their body secretions, particularly saliva through kissing or sharing food utensils. Additionally, patients may continue to be infectious following recovery of their symptoms, as the virus can remain viable in patients for as long as 18 months after the initial infection resolves.

References

1 Filatov, N. and Earle, F.B. (1904). *Semeiology and Diagnosis of Diseases of Children: Together with a Therapeutic Index*, vol. 2, 596. Chicago: Cleveland Press.

2 Sprunt, T.P. and Evans, F.A. (1920). Mononuclear leucocytosis in reaction to acute infections ('infectious mononucleosis'). *Johns Hopkins Hosp Bull* 31: 410–417.

3 Krasteva, A. (2013). Epstein-Barr virus and cytomegalovirus – two herpes viruses with oral manifestations. *J. of IMAB*. 19 (4): 359–362.

4 Balfour, H.H. Jr., Sifakis, F., Sliman, J.A. et al. (2013). Age-specific prevalence of Epstein-Barr virus infection among individuals aged 6–19 years in the United States and factors affecting its acquisition. *J Infect Dis* 208: 1286–1293.

5 Dunmire, S.K., Hogquist, K.A., and Balfour, H.H. (2015). Infectious mononucleosis. *Curr. Top. Microbiol. Immunol.* 390 (Pt 1): 211–240.

6 Vetsika, E. and Callan, M. (2004). Infectious mononucleosis, and Epstein-Barr virus. *Expert Rev. Mol. Med.* 6 (23): 1–16.

7 Marshall-Andon, T. and Heinz, P. (2017). How to use the Monospot and other heterophile antibody tests. *Arch. Dis. Child. Educ. Pract. Ed.* 102 (4): 188–193.

8 Balfour, H.H. Jr., Dunmire, S.K., and Hogquist, K.A. (2015). Infectious mononucleosis. *Clin. Trans. Immunol.* 4: e33.

9 Fugl, A. and Andersen, C.L. (2019). Epstein-Barr virus and its association with disease – a review of relevance to general practice. *BMC Fam. Pract.* 20: 62.

10 Tynell, E., Aurelius, E., Brandell, A. et al. (1996). Acyclovir, and prednisolone treatment of acute infectious mononucleosis: a multicenter, double-blind, placebo-controlled study. *J Infect Dis* 174: 324–331.

11 Luzuriaga, K. and Sullivan, J.L. (2010). Infectious mononucleosis. *N. Engl. J. Med.* 362: 1993–2000.

12 Auwaerter, P.G. (2001). Infectious mononucleosis: return to play. *Clin. Sports Med.* 2004 (23): 485–497.

13 Murray, P.G. and Young, L.S. Epstein-Barr virus infection: basis of malignancy and potential for therapy. *Expert Rev. Mol. Med.* 3 (28): 1–20.

18

Oral Manifestations of Candidosis

Norman Firth[1,2]

[1]University of Queensland, School of Dentistry, Brisbane, Australia
[2]Capital and Coast District Health Board, Wellington, New Zealand

Introduction

Candida species are very common commensal organisms of oral mucosa and may be associated with disease when local or systemic conditions are favourable. Favourable patient factors include either end of the age spectrum and immunosuppression (local or systemic). The most commonly encountered species is *Candida albicans* although carriage rates vary in studies depending on patient factors and methodology [1, 2]. Carriage rates are higher in hospitalised patients compared with ambulant patients.

Oral candidosis is not considered to be a sexually transmitted disease, but it can cause clinical oral manifestations, which are seen in common sexually transmitted diseases and the organism can be transmitted sexually in the absence of active oral mucosal disease.

Epidemiology

Up to 80% of the general population are asymptomatic carriers of *Candida* species; however, carriage is not a reliable predictor of infection. In addition to the oral cavity, the gastrointestinal tract and reproductive tract may have asymptomatic colonisation, and proliferation is controlled by the host immune system and the host microbiotia.

Aetiology and Pathogenesis

C. albicans accounts for approximately 95% of oral candidosis infections. Other species associated with oral candidosis include *Candida parapsilosis*, *Candida tropicalis*, *Candida*

Sexually Transmissible Oral Diseases, First Edition.
Edited by S.R. Prabhu, Nicholas van Wagoner, Jeff Hill and Shailendra Sawleshwarkar.
© 2023 John Wiley & Sons Ltd. Published 2023 by John Wiley & Sons Ltd.

glabrata, *Candida krusei*, *Candida pseudotropicalis*, *Candida guilliermondi* and *Candida dubliniensis* [3, 4]. *C. albicans* is a dimorphic fungus existing in both a yeast phase (blasto-spore, blastoconidial) and a hyphal phase (mycelial). They reproduce by multilateral budding. The environmental conditions determine whether the organism develops in the mycelial yeast form and dimorphism is relevant to both the pathogenicity of the organism and the clinical problems, and aspects related to diagnosis and treatment. Host factors and organism virulence attributes contribute to the pathogenesis of oral candidosis. Local intraoral factors are crucial in the disease process and, therefore, microbial virulence, environmental and host defence factors determine the disease process and clinical manifestations associated with infection [5]. Patients with T-cell-type deficiencies commonly develop candida infections, but these are uncommon in patients with B-cell deficiencies. Susceptibility to oral candida infections may be related to altered T-cell function rather than defects in humoral immunity, whereas prevention of systemic infection is mediated by specific serum antibodies as well as oral effect cells (neutrophils and macrophages) at epithelial sites.

Virulence Factors

In order to cause infection, *Candida* must be retained in the mouth and adhere to mucosal surfaces. Therefore, the washing effects of salivation and swallowing are important factors in host defence against *Candida* growth. Yeasts can adhere to oral epithelium through hydrostatic interactions; attachment is mediated by cell wall receptors, e.g. the agglutin-like sequence family of glycoproteins. Dimorphic growth from yeast to hyphae promotes penetrance of *C. albicans* into tissues and can be considered a virulence factor [6]. Fungi secrete proteolytic enzymes (proteinases and phospholipases), which can cause tissue damage and promote tissue penetrance. Proteinases destroy immunoglobulins and therefore evade the innate immune system. *C. albicans* possesses a group of secreted aspartic proteinases with a range of functions including nutrient acquisition, adhesion, tissue penetration, immune evasion, cell injury following phagocytosis, activation of the blood clotting cascade and enhanced vascular permeability [7].

Clinical Manifestations

A variety of classifications have been proposed since Lehner first published a classification in 1966. The emergence of *Candida* infections in immunocompromised hosts, for example, human immunodeficiency virus (HIV)/acquired immune deficiency syndrome (AIDS) patients and organ transplant recipients lead to a re-think on the classification and changes in terminology.

Pseudomembranous candidosis is frequently called thrush. It is seen in infants, the elderly and the terminally ill [8, 9]. It may be indicative of an underlying serious medical condition. It may also be seen in patients using topical corticosteroid inhalers [10].

Clinically, lesions consist of multiple painless non-adherent white plaques, patches or flecks. Lesions can easily be removed with a blunt instrument leaving an erythematous mucosal base or occasionally a bleeding surface. Affected sites are the soft palate, the oropharynx, tongue, the buccal mucosa and gingiva.

Erythematous candidosis may occur following antibiotic therapy. It has also been termed acute atrophic candidosis or antibiotic sore mouth. Generalised pain may be associated with generalised erythema of the oral mucosa.

A chronic form of erythematous candidosis occurs in the denture bearing area covered by full or partial dentures. This is usually related to poor denture hygiene and failure to remove dentures during sleep. Sharp demarcation between affected erythematous and non-affected mucosal surfaces coinciding with the flange of the denture supports the diagnosis of this form of candidosis [6, 11]. Underlying systemic disease or predisposing factors should be explored, particularly as this form of candidasis is more common in the elderly denture wearing population.

Hyperplastic candidosis is characterised by the presence of irregular white patches and plaques that cannot be scraped off [12]. Diagnosis of this form of candidosis should be confirmed with a biopsy as there is a risk of malignant transformation. Underlying systemic disease and predisposing factors together with risk factors for oral candidosis should be addressed.

Angular cheilitis, characterised by erythema and cracking at the angles of the mouth, may be associated with both *Candida* and bacterial infection [13]. Underlying systemic disease and predisposing factors have a role to play and should be investigated.

Median rhomboid glossitis presenting as an erythematous atrophic lesion on the dorsum of the tongue near the junction of the anterior two thirds and posterior third is also considered to be related to candidal infection [14]. Lesions may be speckled or nodular, and a biopsy may be required to confirm the diagnosis if the lesion is clinically suspicious of malignancy.

Concomitant candidosis occurs in association with other oral mucosal lesions, for example lichen planus, chronic ulceration (Figure 18.1a,b, and c) or keratoses (with or without epithelial dysplasia) (Figure 18.2a,b, and c) and require treatment in addition to the usual management of other oral lesions. An additional biopsy following antifungal treatment is frequently required particularly if epithelial dysplasia is present.

Medical conditions in which oral, perioral, generalised or systemic candidosis occur include candidosis endocrinopathy syndrome, diffuse chronic mucocutaneous candidosis, familial chronic mucocutaneous candidosis, Di-George syndrome and HIV/AIDS. Patients undergoing radiotherapy for head and neck cancer are susceptible to candidosis during and post-treatment.

Haematological investigations are important in assessing possible underlying predisposing factors including iron, vitamin B12 or folate deficiency, or an undiagnosed or poorly controlled diabetes mellitus.

Diagnosis is often based on clinical findings alone; however, as indicated above, biopsy may be indicated [15]. Smears can be stained with periodic acid-Schiff (PAS) or potassium hydroxide (KOH), and this may provide quick confirmation of diagnosis in clinical settings where the facilities are available [5, 14].

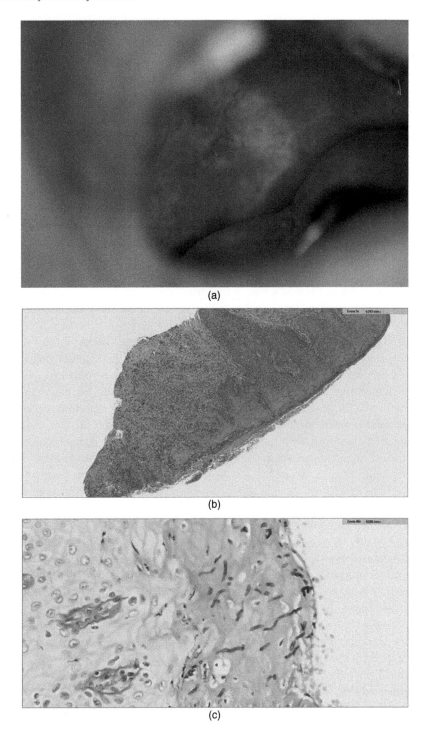

(a)

(b)

(c)

Figure 18.1 (a)–(c) A woman aged 57 years with non-healing ulcer of four weeks duration on the soft palate. (a) Source: Clinical photograph kindly provided by Dr. Jacinta Vu, Oral Medicine Specialist, Perth Oral Medicine & Dental Sleep Centre. (b) Photomicrograph showing non-specific ulceration with no features of epithelial dysplasia or malignancy (H&E). (c) Photomicrograph showing *Candida* hyphae in the epithelium adjacent the region of ulceration (PAS-D) 165913-21CL.

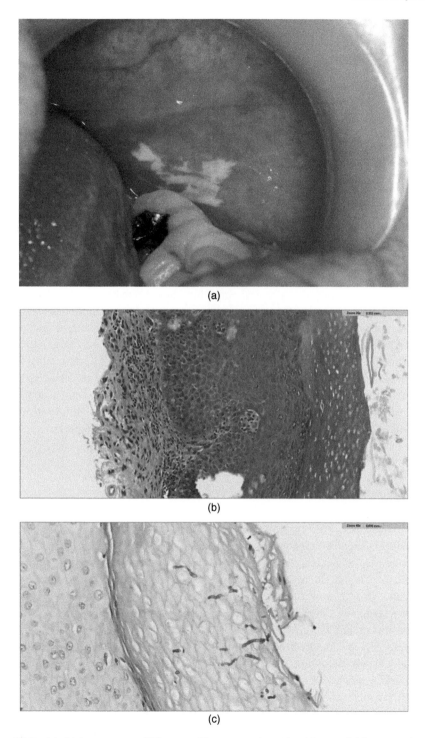

(a)

(b)

(c)

Figure 18.2 (a)–(c) A woman aged 78 years with an asymptomatic white patch/plaque on the left buccal mucosa. Source: (a) Clinical photograph kindly provided by Dr. Amanda Phoon Nguyen, Oral Medicine Specialist, Perth Oral Medicine & Dental Sleep Centre. (b) Photomicrograph showing thick orthokeratin, mild epithelial dysplasia in the absence of significant epithelial hyperplasia (H&E). (c) Photomicrograph showing *Candida* hyphae in the orthokeratin (PAS-D). 165903-21CL.

Treatment

Topical treatment of oral candid infections is usually effective. Two polyenes have been used since the 1950s and are still used today. These agents are nystatin and amphotericin B. Nystatin is toxic and cannot be administered parenterally nor is it absorbed from the gastrointestinal tract and, therefore, is restricted to topical use only. A variety of forms including cream, ointment, tablets, suspension, gel, pessary and pastille are available, but not all are available in all countries. Amphotericin B is not well absorbed from the gastrointestinal tract and is used topically (for localised) or intravenously (for systemic infection). Lozenges are commonly used in conjunction with a nystatin preparation. The tongue is a reservoir for candida and the value of lozenges cannot be underestimated. Adjunctive measures including antiseptic mouth rinses, for example, chlorhexidine gluconate for oral and denture hygiene might be useful and sialagogues for patients with hyposalivation should be considered [16].

For over 30 years, imidazoles and triazoles have been used in the treatment of oral candidal infections. These agents include miconazole, clotrimazole, fluconazole and itraconazole. Miconazole is useful as a topical agent but should not be used in patients taking warfarin as it potentiates the effect of warfarin with potentially fatal consequences. Possible side effects of systemically administered antifungals should be considered, and this may preclude their use in some patients. Ketoconazole, for example, is associated with hepatotoxicity and is no longer commercially available. The emergence of antimicrobial resistant strains of candida is also an issue encountered when antifungal agents including fluconazole were administered prophylactically to HIV/AIDS patients. The echinocandin caspofungin administered intravenously is effective in managing patients with invasive candidosis or candidaemia with a fewer side effects then parenterally administered amphotericin B [17].

References

1 McCullough, M.J., Clemons, K.V., and Stevens, D.A. (1999). Molecular epidemiology of the global and temporal diversity of *Candida albicans*. *Clin. Infect. Dis.* 29: 1220–1225.

2 Reichart, P.A., Samaranayake, L.P., and Philipsen, H.P. (2000). Pathology and clinical correlates in oral candidiasis and its variants: a review. *Oral Dis.* 6: 85–91.

3 McCullough, M.J., Ross, B.C., and Reade, P.C. (1996). *Candida albicans*: a review of its history, taxonomy, epidemiology, virulence attributes, and methods of strain differentiation. *Int. J. Oral Maxillofac. Surg.* 25: 136–144.

4 Al-Karaawi, Z.M., Manfredi, M., Waugh, A.C. et al. (2002). Molecular characterization of Candida spp. isolated from the oral cavities of patients from diverse clinical settings. *Oral Microbiol. Immunol.* 17: 44–49.

5 Farah, C.S., Ashman, R.B., and Challacombe, S.J. (2000). Oral candidiasis. *Clin. Dermatol.* 18: 553–562. https://doi.org/10.1016/s0738-081x(00)00145-0.

6 Farah, C.S., Lynch, N., and McCullough, M.J. (2010). Oral fungal infections: an update for the general practitioner. *Aust. Dent. J.* 55 (Suppl 1): 48–54.

7 Cannon, R.D., Holmes, A.R., and Firth, N.A. (2019). Chapter 17. Fungi and fungal infections of the oral cavity. In: *Oral Microbiology and Immunology*, 3e (ed. R.J. Lamont, G.N. Hajishengallis, H.M. Koo and H.F. Jenkinson). ASM https://doi.org/10.1128/9781555 819996.

8 Muzyka, B.C. (2005). Oral fungal infections. *Dent. Clin. N. Am.* 49: 49–65.viii.

9 Patton, L.L. (2013). Oral lesions associated with human immunodeficiency virus disease. *Dent. Clin. N. Am.* 57: 673–698.

10 Ellepola, A.N. and Samaranayake, L.P. (2001). Inhalational and topical steroids, and oral candidiasis: a mini review. *Oral Dis.* 7: 211–216.

11 Arendorf, T.M. and Walker, D.M. (1987). Denture stomatitis: a review. *J. Oral Rehabil.* 14: 217–227.

12 McCullough, M.J. and Savage, N.W. (2005). Oral candidiasis and the therapeutic use of antifungal agents in dentistry. *Aust. Dent. J.* 50: S36–S39.

13 Wilkieson, C., Samaranayake, L.P., MacFarlane, T.W. et al. (1991). Oral candidiasis in the elderly in long term hospital care. *J. Oral Pathol. Med.* 20: 13–16.

14 Akpan, A. and Morgan, R. (2002). Oral candidiasis. *Postgrad. Med. J.* 78: 455–459.

15 Williams, D.W. and Lewis, M.A. (2000). Isolation and identification of Candida from the oral cavity. *Oral Dis.* 6: 3–11.

16 Lalla, R.V. and Dongari-Bagtzoglou, A. (2014). Antifungal medications or disinfectants for denture stomatitis. *Evid. Based Dent.* 15 (2): 61–62. https://doi.org/10.1038/sj.ebd.6401032.

17 Lakshman, P., Samaranayake, L.P., Keung Leung, W., and Jin, L. (2009). Oral mucosal fungal infections. *Periodontol 2000.* 49 (1): 39–59. https://doi.org/10.1111/j.1600-0757. 2008.00291.x.

Index

Sexually Transmissible Oral Diseases, First Edition.
Edited by S.R. Prabhu, Nicholas van Wagoner, Jeff Hill and Shailendra Sawleshwarkar.
© 2023 John Wiley & Sons Ltd. Published 2023 by John Wiley & Sons Ltd.